BIRTH IN TIMES OF DESPAIR

ANTHROPOLOGIES OF AMERICAN MEDICINE: CULTURE, POWER, AND PRACTICE

General Editors: Paul Brodwin, Michele Rivkin-Fish, and Susan Shaw

Transnational Reproduction: Race, Kinship, and Commercial Surrogacy in India
Daisy Deomampo

Unequal Coverage: The Experience of Health Care Reform in the United States
Edited by Jessica Mulligan and Heide Castañeda

The New American Servitude: Political Belonging among African Immigrant Home Care Workers
Cati Coe

War and Health: The Medical Consequences of the Wars in Iraq and Afghanistan
Catherine Lutz and Andrea Mazzarino

Inequalities of Aging: Paradoxes of Independence in American Home Care
Elana D. Buch

Reproductive Injustice: Racism, Pregnancy, and Premature Birth
Dána-Ain Davis

Living on the Spectrum: Autism and Youth in Community
Elizabeth Fein

Adverse Events: Race, Inequality, and the Testing of New Pharmaceuticals
Jill A. Fisher

Motherhood on Ice: The Mating Gap and Why Women Freeze Their Eggs
Marcia C. Inhorn

Violence that Never Heals: The Lifelong Effects of Intimate Partner Violence for Immigrant Women
Allison Bloom

Conceiving Christian America: The Reproductive Politics of White Saviorism in Embryo Adoption
Risa Cromer

Pregnant at Work: Low-Wage Workers, Power, and Temporal Injustice
Elise Andaya

Good Intentions in Global Health: Medical Missions, Emotion, and Health Care across Borders
Nicole S. Berry

Birth in Times of Despair: Reproductive Violence on the US-Mexico Border
Carina Heckert

Birth in Times of Despair

Reproductive Violence on the US-Mexico Border

Carina Heckert

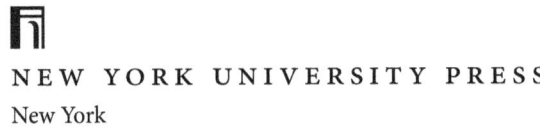

NEW YORK UNIVERSITY PRESS
New York

NEW YORK UNIVERSITY PRESS
New York
www.nyupress.org

© 2024 by New York University
All rights reserved

Please contact the Library of Congress for Cataloging-in-Publication data.
ISBN: 9781479832064 (hardback)
ISBN: 9781479832071 (paperback)
ISBN: 9781479832101 (library ebook)
ISBN: 9781479832095 (consumer ebook)

This book is printed on acid-free paper, and its binding materials are chosen for strength and durability. We strive to use environmentally responsible suppliers and materials to the greatest extent possible in publishing our books.

Manufactured in the United States of America

10 9 8 7 6 5 4 3 2 1

Also available as an ebook

For Gabito, my pandemic baby.

CONTENTS

Introduction: *Desesperación*	1
1. Legislating Maternal Harm	39
2. Immigration Policy and Embodied Vulnerabilities	67
3. The Local Biology of Preeclampsia	89
4. Conjugated Harm and Pregnancy during the Pandemic	114
5. Finding Compassionate Care	134
6. Navigating *Impotencia* during the Postpartum Period	161
Conclusion: Imagining Reproductive Justice in the Borderlands	181
Acknowledgments	193
Appendix I: Integrating Cortisol Testing into Ethnographic Research	197
Appendix II: Participant Characteristics	203
Appendix III: Emotional Distress and Health Vulnerabilities	205
Notes	209
Bibliography	217
Index	239
About the Author	247

Introduction

Desesperación

"If I go outside, I feel that *desesperación* [despair]. It's like this worry and an anxiety. I feel this despair in my hands and my feet," Brisa, an undocumented immigrant from rural Mexico, explained. She went on to name the primary causes of this despair: the constant reminders of immigration enforcement in the US-Mexico border city of El Paso, Texas, and her economic precarity. These two factors were inseparable. Brisa had borrowed thousands of dollars from a distant family member to migrate to the United States in early 2019. By late 2020, at the time of our first interview, Brisa had paused making payments on the loan and was receiving frequent, threatening messages from the woman who had lent her the money. Each message left Brisa with feelings of despair and powerlessness, as she did not have a source of steady income. She had lost most of her jobs cleaning houses in March 2020, when stay-at-home orders in response to the COVID-19 pandemic went into effect. Although she tried desperately to find other work, the combination of her immigration status, the pandemic, and becoming pregnant made it difficult to secure a job. She expressed intense worry over returning to cleaning houses, fearful that frequent exposure to cleaning products could harm the baby. A recent miscarriage had heightened this concern. In the summer of 2020, she had an interview at a restaurant that allowed servers to work off-the-books, earning only tips. When she arrived to the interview, US Border Patrol agents were dining. In the US-Mexico border region, seeing immigration officials is an inescapable part of daily life. These encounters may be experienced as intense stress for local residents, even those who are US-born citizens (Sabo et al. 2014). Given the insecurities Brisa felt over her immigration status, she knew she could not work at that restaurant if immigration officials would be regular customers. She said of the incident, "I felt panicked, almost like I couldn't breathe. I wanted to leave right away."

Brisa was thirty-four-weeks pregnant when we first spoke and she repeated the theme of *desesperación* as she named various discomforts she was experiencing. She described the swelling in her hands and feet as a feeling of *desesperación*. Swelling can also be a symptom of preeclampsia, a condition in which there is a disruption to the blood supply between the pregnant person[1] and the fetus. It can lead to a sudden rise in blood pressure and damage major organs, especially the liver and kidneys. Without medical intervention, it can become life threatening, making it a leading cause of maternal mortality and morbidity (Roberts and Bell 2013). Brisa's midwife did in fact diagnose her with preeclampsia at her next prenatal visit. The preeclampsia had already become severe, and Brisa consented to her midwife's recommendation to induce labor. The pregnancy and birth included a number of other complications, including gestational diabetes, a retained placenta that required manual removal, and postpartum hemorrhage. After a four-day hospital stay, Brisa went home, only to return to the emergency room days later. She explained, "After leaving the hospital, I got worse. I started feeling the high blood pressure again. They [doctors in the ER] gave me medicine that worked after a few hours and my body, my feet, the swelling was going down, and I felt like the headache was gone." The headache that Brisa experienced is another telltale sign of preeclampsia. Given that preeclampsia is related to blood flow to and from the placenta, symptoms of the condition typically resolve postpartum. However, postpartum preeclampsia can occur weeks following delivery, even for a person who did not have preeclampsia during the pregnancy (Yancey et al. 2011). Brisa's postpartum preeclampsia could have become life-threatening had she not returned to the hospital. Postpartum health challenges continued for Brisa. At her only postpartum checkup, her provider informed her that she had postpartum depression based on a questionnaire she filled out.

Despair, the most common translation for *desesperación*, does not fully capture what this emotion entails and how Brisa experienced it. As Brisa points out, her *desesperación* was the product of social circumstances beyond her control. Brisa and other women often referenced this emotion in relation to a feeling of *impotencia*, or powerlessness. *Desesperación* also includes the bodily effects resulting from one's mental state. According to Kurt Organista and colleagues (2016), *desesperación* is an idiom of distress that immigrant Latinos may evoke when migration goals have been thrown off course and health ailments follow. The symptoms of *desesperación* often overlap with anxiety and depression but also include distinct emotions such as feeling overwhelmed, angsty, and frustrated (Organista, Arreola, and Neilands 2016). According to Brisa, her *desesperación* caused the bodily sensations she felt as she developed preeclampsia.

In Brisa's case, the pandemic upended her ability to work and exacerbated the precariousness she felt from being undocumented. When Brisa borrowed money from a distant family member living in San Antonio, Texas, the funds enabled her to pay off her previous debts that she had incurred in her hometown during periods of economic hardship. With suppressed wages in Mexico, she had been unable to repay those loans. Brisa also used the borrowed money to travel to Mexico's northern border and with a relative's identity documents crossed into the United States and made her way to San Antonio to be with her mother and several siblings, all of whom had been residing in the United States for years. Her hope was to finally achieve economic stability through higher wages in the United States. What she referred to as her "life project" of economic independence remained elusive as the combination of her immigration status, the pandemic, and her pregnancy limited her ability to earn money. Initially, she lived and worked in San Antonio, with her family connections providing an important source of social support. As the pandemic led her to lose most of her income, she became uncomfortable with the constant requests from relatives to repay her loan. The pressure became enough to spur Brisa to relocate over five hundred miles to El Paso, Texas. In El Paso, she lived with a friend in view of the border fence and frequent sightings of Border Patrol trucks and helicopters. At the time, she was also navigating a complicated romantic relationship, which resulted in two pregnancies. The first pregnancy ended in miscarriage, while the second resulted in the birth of her daughter. During our first interview, while she was still pregnant, Brisa was uncertain about whether she wanted to continue her relationship with the father. Concerned that he was not ready for parenthood, she had decided to distance herself from him. Yet after the birth, she made the decision to marry the father in hopes that this arrangement would offer her more stability, including the option to stay home with the baby as opposed to quickly returning to work and having to leave her newborn at a daycare in the middle of a pandemic. Brisa's *desesperación* was a product of her social world and shaped and constrained her decisions about her intimate life. While she was happy about being able to have time with the baby, not working continued to prevent her from repaying her loan, leading to continued despair.

Brisa's frequent reference to feelings of *desesperación* as a cause of ill health both during her pregnancy and postpartum reflects a larger theme that shapes the focus of this book. This book interrogates experiences of pregnancy, birth, and the postpartum period in the border city of El Paso, which has been a symbolic battleground in the enactment of immigration and border policies, experienced a racially motivated mass shooting in 2019, and faced particular challenges due to the COVID-19 pandemic. It traces the ripple effects of these social stressors within the community, even for people who have not been directly impacted by these specific events, and particularly for those whose pregnancies overlapped with these key moments. I argue that the social and emotional toll produced by the multipronged experiences of unjust immigration policies, a lack of gun control, a business-driven health care system that fails vulnerable populations, and legislative efforts to control reproduction contributes to adverse maternal and infant health outcomes and should be considered a form of reproductive violence.

Much of this volume draws on interviews conducted as part of multiple projects on maternal health and emotional distress in the context of overlapping crises in the US-Mexico border region. These projects took place in 2018–19 and 2020–22. From August 2018 to May 2019, I led a project that involved interviews with thirty-five pregnant and postpartum first- and second-generation immigrants in El Paso. Escalating threats of immigration enforcement under the Donald Trump administration characterized this time. The effects of immigration policies are particularly profound in border communities as the region serves as a symbolic battleground in politicized debates and the public imaginary. Given the significant anxiety and uncertainty surrounding immigration policy, we focused on the role of immigration concerns as they related to the emotional experience of pregnancy and the postpartum period.

Beginning in September 2020, I began a larger scale interdisciplinary project that continued to focus on emotional distress and maternal health. I maintained a focus on immigration-related concerns, but given the COVID-19 pandemic, I expanded the scope of the research to capture the social and mental health toll of the pandemic. At the time, El Paso was still recovering from one of the deadliest mass shootings in US history, an act driven by racist and anti-immigrant sentiment. Thus, instead of focusing only on first- and second-generation immigrants, we included Latinas with a range of citizenship and immigration histories to further explore the community effects of immigration policy, anti-immigrant sentiment, and the racism and various forms of violence experienced within border communities. By including both US-born citizens as well as foreign-born women, I focus on the ways immigration policy generates harm, and not just for those with a precarious immigrations status. Immigration concerns go beyond one's own immigration status, as connections to others—partners, siblings, parents, extended family members, and friends—profoundly influence a person's emotional well-being. This project included colleagues in sociology, women and gender studies, neuroscience, and obstetrics and gynecology. With a sample of 176 Latinas utilizing publicly funded care and recruited from a clinical context, we collected survey data, health records, and cortisol samples from hair (a biomarker for stress), enabling us to compare self-reported experiences of stress to stress-sensitive health outcomes and physiological biomarkers of stress. We conducted in-depth interviews with a subsample of sixty of these women and conducted multiple interviews with fourteen of them throughout the first year postpartum. This project began toward the beginning of the public health, social, and economic crises generated by the COVID-19 pandemic and continued as the pandemic evolved. This book therefore is able to offer insights drawing on a rare methodological integration of biocultural and ethnographic approaches.

Like Brisa, many of the people interviewed for this book described how sociopolitical events created a sense of despair and how they felt that their resulting emotions had negative consequences for their health and the health of their babies. While women often situated their narrative in relation to recent events, especially the hardships created by the pandemic, these experiences are the product of persistent and long-standing inequities experienced by border residents. Women often described an array of emotions during pregnancy and the postpartum period, including happiness over having a child. The repeated theme of despair reflects the disempowering social and political contexts that at times constrained women's agency and limited their ability to have and raise a child in the conditions that they desired. The despair that has characterized the backdrop of pregnancy and postpartum experiences is ultimately about failed policies: unjust immigration policies, stalled legislation for gun regulations, a business-driven health care model that has become too expensive and inaccessible in times of health crises, inadequate public safety nets, and legislative efforts to control reproduction.

Combined failures in multiple policy realms created a sense of *desesperación* for Brisa and many others who participated in this research. Despite this despair, women also often professed feelings of joy. Brisa was happy about her pregnancy and becoming a mother. Her despair came from the ways that policies limited her ability to be a mother in the ways that she desired. Her desires were fundamental: a life without fear of being deported and forced to choose whether to take her child with her for the sake of family unity or leave her without a mother in a country where she would have more opportunities; access to a basic level of health care that would ensure she could seek services without going into further debt; and the availability of a social safety net so that she would not feel crippled by economic anxiety during a time when she faced an impossible choice of whether or not to return to work and leave her newborn in daycare in the middle of a pandemic. Brisa's account shows how policy decisions that limit the abilities of individuals, families, and communities to thrive produced despair that clouded her happiness over becoming a mother. Those experiencing multiple domains of oppression related to gender, immigration status, race and ethnicity, and socioeconomic status disproportionately feel this burden.

The Maternal Harm of Health and Immigration Policies

Most maternal deaths are preventable. When deaths occur, it is often a reflection of social inequities and faults in the health care system that impede a timely diagnosis and care, through either a blatant denial of optimal care or providers failing to listen to birthing and postpartum individuals' reports of concerning symptoms (Declercq and Zephyrin 2020). MacDorman and colleagues published a 2016 article with a finding that from 2010 to 2012, the maternal mortality rate in Texas had doubled. The article concluded by saying that "in the absence of war, natural disaster, or economic upheaval, the doubling of a mortality rate within a 2-year period . . . seems unlikely." A subsequent state-specific analysis pointed to a less alarming increase, as potential reporting errors had led to poor data (MacDorman et al. 2018). However, it is clear that the maternal mortality rate has been rising in Texas and that the rate is disproportionately high for minorities and those residing in rural locations and border counties. Additionally, the Texas Maternal Mortality and Morbidity Task Force (Texas DSHS 2018) found that 56 percent of maternal deaths occur more than sixty days postpartum and that maternal deaths in the extended postpartum period may go underreported, in large part because of the inaccessibility of care. While this book is not specifically about maternal deaths, the maternal mortality rate in the United States—which is the highest of all industrialized countries—is indicative of a deeper maternal health crisis, especially among people of color (MacDorman et al. 2021).

The maternal mortality rate is a single measure that does not fully capture experiences of harm that may occur throughout the trajectory of pregnancy, birth, and the postpartum period. While data captured at the time of birth, especially low birthweight, preterm birth, and infant deaths, are well documented, there is poor tracking of the less quantifiable experiences of harm that may come in the form of traumatic birth experiences, postpartum depression, unsuccessful attempts of breastfeeding, and social and economic crises resulting from a lack of employment and other protections for new parents.

One factor contributing to maternal harm is the inaccessibility of health services, especially postpartum. In part because Texas did not expand Medicaid under the Affordable Care Act (ACA), the state has the highest uninsured rate in the country (Texas Medical Association 2016), with higher uninsured rates in border counties than nonborder counties. The uninsured rate among the population under age sixty-five is 26 percent in El Paso County (Buettgens, Blumberg, and Pan 2018). Women of reproductive age have an especially high uninsured rate but may qualify for a publicly funded program during pregnancy. What program a person has access to is contingent on their immigration status.

Health Policy as Immigration Policy

Immigration policies have significant bearing on a person's ability to access health care. Undocumented immigrants are less likely than US citizens and permanent residents to hold jobs that offer access to private health insurance (Artiga and Diaz 2019) and immigration status factors into eligibility criteria for publicly funded health programs. Notably, undocumented immigrants and permanent residents with less than five years of legal residency do not qualify for Texas Medicaid programs.[2] Undocumented immigrants and those with Deferred Action for Childhood Arrivals (DACA) also do not qualify for federal subsidies under the ACA. These exclusionary policies have ripple effects, as citizen members of mixed-status families fear the implications of what their use of public programs might mean for undocumented family members (Castañeda 2018).

Elise Andaya describes pregnancy as a "temporary zone of inclusion" (2018, 105), as it is a time when those who are otherwise uninsured may qualify for publicly funded programs. However, this inclusion is partial and unequitable for immigrants, with policies varying by state. At the time of my research, Texas Medicaid for Pregnant Women provided comprehensive coverage for lower income individuals during pregnancy until two months postpartum. However, federal Medicaid funding is limited to US citizens and qualified legal residents although some states have used various mechanisms to expand coverage to precariously documented immigrants.[3] Texas is one of twenty states that offers publicly funded prenatal coverage to precariously documented immigrants and recent legal residents through the Children's Health Insurance Program (CHIP) Perinatal provisions. However, coverage under Texas CHIP Perinatal is extremely limited, covering only prenatal appointments, delivery, and up to two postpartum visits. Care is not comprehensive and covered expenses include only a limited range of conditions defined as posing a risk to the fetus. Brisa's return visit to the emergency room, for example, was not covered by CHIP Perinatal. Even though postpartum preeclampsia can be life-threatening, it did not pose a physical risk to her US-citizen baby. When Brisa went to her only postpartum appointment covered under the program, she was told she may have postpartum depression. Since CHIP Perinatal would not cover follow-up treatment for postpartum depression, she received a referral to a community clinic. Other interlocutors reported significant health and economic struggles because they suffered conditions not covered under CHIP Perinatal. For example, Rita was an undocumented woman who had recently left an abusive relationship. After giving birth to twins via C-section, her incision reopened and required surgery. Since the surgery was separate from the prenatal care and delivery covered by CHIP Perinatal, she was responsible for paying for the procedure. Other conditions that interlocutors lacked coverage for under CHIP Perinatal included hospitalization for COVID-19, a urinary tract infection, false labor, and diagnostic tests that assist providers with the management of preexisting hypertension. If left unmanaged, such health conditions can generate riskier pregnancies (Bingham, Strauss, and Coeytaux 2011). This inequitable access to care as it relates to immigration status can be a significant source of maternal harm.

Beyond the limited scope of CHIP Perinatal, some people choose not to apply for this program out of fear over the consequences of utilizing public benefits. Hesitations in applying for CHIP Perinatal were especially pronounced during the Trump administration. In October 2018, the Trump administration announced planned changes to the "likely public charge" rule, which immigration officials can use to deny immigration petitions on the grounds that an applicant would likely use publicly funded programs. Between 1996 and 2018, United States Citizenship and Immigration Services (USCIS) guidelines stated that use of noncash public benefits, such as health and nutrition programs, would not cause an applicant to be labeled a likely public charge. While the Trump administration announced plans to expand the definition of likely public charge in October 2018, the updated protocol was not released until August 2019, leaving a nearly one-year period when there was significant uncertainty over which programs would lead a person to be labeled a likely public charge. The new guidelines did allow for use of publicly funded prenatal care and nutrition programs under the Women, Infants, and Children (WIC) program. However, during our interviews that took place from 2018 to 2019, pregnant people and service providers alike expressed uncertainty over how use of CHIP Perinatal and WIC could impact future immigration applications such as green card renewals, adjustment of status, and naturalization. Epidemiological evidence suggests widespread negative health ramifications as a consequence of the enactment of immigration policies under the Trump administration (Williams and Medlock 2017; Woolhandler et al. 2021). Underutilization of prenatal care as a consequence of fearing to use CHIP Perinatal is one of the ways that political threats aimed at immigrants translated into potentially adverse health outcomes.[4]

Racialization and Immigration Policy in the Border Region

The trajectory of the likely public charge rule highlights the extent to which immigration policies have been used to exclude racialized populations. Women, and particularly Asians and Latinas, have historically faced exclusions as a mechanism for deterring reproduction and permanent resettlement among their male counterparts (Chavez 2008; Park 2011). Beginning with the Page Act of 1875, immigration laws established protocols for denying entry of and deporting individuals who were likely public charges due to ill health or disability. The act aimed to exclude Chinese immigrants and used medical racism to achieve this goal. The American Medical Association played a critical role in supporting this legislation by claiming Chinese people carried exotic germs that could threaten white people. Enforcement of the act soon expanded to the US-Mexico border, primarily because Mexican laborers had been constructed as socially undesirable and as vectors of infection (Molina 2011). In the decades following the Page Act, immigration officials routinely used the likely public charge rule to deny entry to pregnant women and deport pregnant immigrants (Park 2011).

Exclusionary policies related to the perceived health of immigrants go beyond the likely public charge rule. The passage of immigration reform and welfare reform in 1996 included changes aimed at further excluding immigrants from social programs, with harmful repercussions for maternal health. Before 1996, authorized immigrants had the same degree of access as citizens to public safety-net programs such as Medicaid. The passage of welfare reform included length of residency requirements for immigrants to receive public benefits, which was largely a reflection of public discourse that perceived reproduction among immigrants as a drain on public resources (Chavez 2008). California highlights the impact these reforms had on pregnant immigrants, as policy changes led to the state dropping seventy thousand individuals from state-sponsored prenatal coverage (Park 2011).

The US government has also historically weaponized immigration policy to delegitimize US citizens of Mexican heritage. This history includes deportation campaigns during the Great Depression that resulted in the removal of an estimated one to two million US citizens of Mexican ancestry. Welfare offices and hospitals throughout the Southwest were complicit in turning over the information of Mexican clients (Balderrama and Rodríguez 2006). Beginning in 1928, the county hospital in El Paso began reporting Mexican patients, including US citizens, to immigration authorities. This pattern points to how US policies have treated "Mexican" as an identity of perpetual foreignness, justifying various forms of exclusion of US-born citizens of Mexican descent (Sinclair 2016).

More subtle forms of delegitimizing the citizenship status of the children of immigrants persist, especially in Texas, where there have been systematic efforts to deny birth certificates and passports to US-born citizens with noncitizen parents. For example, Itzel is a US-born citizen who gave birth to her fourth child in the spring of 2021. Her mother was a Mexican citizen who came to El Paso for the birth. Itzel was born in 1992 in a birth center run by midwives in El Paso—a detail that she believes has prevented her from being able to obtain a US passport. This is a part of a larger pattern of the US State Department denying passports to Latino border residents who had their birth registered with a midwife outside of a hospital context. In the 1990s, there was evidence that a small number of midwives in Texas border counties had falsely registered some births as taking place in the United States. Beginning under the George W. Bush administration, those cases served as a pretext to question the citizenship of thousands of US-born citizens who were delivered outside of a hospital setting. Subsequent administrations continued with these passport denials, and overall denials to Latinos appeared to spike under the Trump administration (Sieff 2018). When Itzel applied for a passport, she was asked to provide additional evidence of the circumstances of her birth. When she sought legal advice, a lawyer informed her it would cost approximately $10,000 to fight her case—a sum of money she did not have. To be clear, Itzel had a US birth certificate and was able to secure other identity documents that are normally required to prove citizenship. It was only a US passport, key for her mobility across the border, which she could not obtain.

More recently, in 2013, Texas began restricting the types of documents that parents could use to prove their own identities when applying for a birth certificate for their child. Most significantly, the state stopped accepting consular IDs and foreign passports without a valid visa as acceptable identity documents. The required types of identity documents were often impossible for undocumented individuals to obtain, leading to the systematic denial of birth certificates to US-born citizens with undocumented parents. Without a birth certificate, parents may be unable to prove their relationship to a US-citizen child, creating obstacles for school enrollment and accessing public health programs. Texas's efforts to restrict undocumented parents from obtaining birth certificates offers a clear example of how immigration policies disenfranchise US citizens (Castañeda 2019). These restrictions for obtaining birth certificates persisted until 2016, when a legal settlement resulted in the expansion of the types of IDs that parents could use to secure a child's birth certificate.

Beyond such procedural efforts, over the past several decades there have been numerous congressional bills aimed at ending birthright citizenship. Such efforts rely on discourses of a "Hispanic invasion" and assumptions that pregnant immigrants are coming to the United States for the purpose of birthing US citizens who will then utilize publicly funded programs (Chavez 2017). As Leo Chavez (2017) points out, the term "anchor baby" fuels these legislative efforts while delegitimizing the citizenship status of US-born children of immigrants. Such patterns reflect how the US government has historically treated people of Latino ancestry as what Mae Ngai (2006) dubs "alien citizens."

During the Trump administration, threats of workplace raids and massive deportation campaigns generated fears not just for the undocumented but also for their family members and broader communities. While militarization of the US-Mexico border has long relied on racist imagery (Díaz-Barriga and Dorsey 2020), the Trump administration amplified these racial undertones. This was particularly evident through the enactment of draconian policies aimed to prevent primarily Brown asylum seekers at the US-Mexico border from entering the United States. Such policies included Zero Tolerance (2018), which separated children from their parents, and the Migrant Protection Protocols (2019), which denied asylum seekers entry to the United States until they received a court date. The Trump administration justified these policies under a discourse that framed asylum seekers as invading the country, ignoring the fact that from 2016 to 2020, apprehensions at the US-Mexico border were at the lowest point since the mid-1970s, with the exception of a spike in 2019 (American Immigration Council 2022). In early 2020, the Centers for Disease Control and Prevention (CDC), under the authority of the Trump administration, used the COVID-19 public health emergency as justification to invoke Title 42, an obscure public health provision that allows the federal government to restrict the entry of foreigners to limit the spread of a communicable disease. The Trump administration used Title 42 to override US and international asylum law, forcing asylum seekers to remain in Mexico. Subsequent investigative reporting has shown that this measure was never about public health. Instead, the Trump administration capitalized on the pandemic to further a racialized anti-immigrant agenda (Dickerson and Shear 2020). The Joe Biden administration delayed ending this policy, and when it did propose an end to Title 42, court decisions kept the measure in place until the end of the public health emergency in May 2023. Between 2020 and 2023, there were periods with significant increases in migrants attempting to enter the United States. The political and economic turmoil unleashed by the pandemic combined with years of limited routes for requesting asylum contributed to this pattern (American Immigration Council 2022). The political response has involved further militarization of border communities and continued exclusionary responses to asylum seekers.

Given that El Paso serves as a transitional zone, as asylum seekers released by immigration authorities tend to leave the city for other destinations, we interviewed very few people who were in the process of seeking asylum or who had family members seeking asylum. However, in a city with strong cross-border ties, most people at least have extended family members who were foreign-born and tend to view the inhumane treatment of asylum seekers as a part of a broader anti-immigrant agenda. Further, the racist undertones of anti-immigrant sentiment are acutely felt in a community where 82.9 percent of the population identifies as Hispanic or Latino (US Census Bureau 2021).

The State of Texas has used the increase in migrants at the US-Mexico border to enact its own agenda to further militarize the region. In March 2021, the state reappropriated Operation Border Health Preparedness, an aid program that provided medical and dental services in border counties, to create Operation Lone Star. Operation Lone Star diverted state funding to station more law enforcement agents and the National Guard at the border. This shift took funds away from public health in a medically underserved region during a pandemic to finance border militarization (see Lucas, Castañeda, and Melo 2023). Given the familial and other affective ties that connect US citizens to noncitizens, border militarization and immigration policies have spillover effects. Deportations and detention produce social, emotional, and economic hardships for families and their broader communities (Boehm 2012; Castañeda 2019; Dreby 2015; Lopez 2019). It is not just the events of deportation and detention themselves but also anticipation and memories experienced at both the individual and collective level that can serve as a source of trauma (Talavera, Núñez-Mchiri, and Heyman 2010).

While race has always been fundamental to the enactment of US immigration policy, social constructions of race are complex and uneven, especially in the border region. The border region was once Mexico, prior to the 1848 Treaty of Hidalgo that resulted in Mexico ceding 55 percent of its territory to the Unites States. As white settlers increasingly encroached in on the region, "American" emerged as a racial category to distinguish Anglos from people of Mexican descent, many of whom were US citizens. "Mexican" came to signify perpetual foreignness, even for US citizens of Mexican descent (Sinclair 2016). The racialization of Mexicans goes beyond nationality and citizenship, as social class and skin color have factored into how Anglos treated and interacted with those they labeled as Mexicans. Telling is the legacy of disinfection stations, or "bath houses," at US ports of entry. Bath houses were a part of border health posts from 1917 to 1960. Individuals whom border authorities determined to be a potential public health risk were sent for delousing and disinfection using Zyklon B and DDT. As historian David Romo (2005) uncovered, Zyklon B was a chemical later used in the Nazi death camps, and high-ranking Nazis praised the use of this disinfection

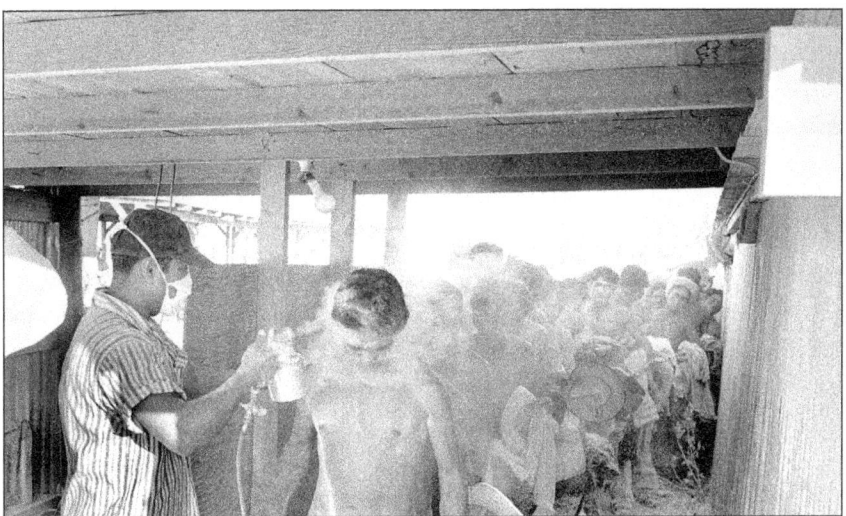

Figure I.1: Border crossers having DDT sprayed in their faces at a border health post, 1956
Credit: Leonard Nadel, courtesy National Museum of American History

strategy on the border. The inconsistencies in whom authorities sent for disinfection reveal how border policies were less about nationality than about race and social class. Many of those labeled "Mexican" were US citizens. It was their poverty and phenotype that typically led them to be sent for disinfection. Conversely, wealthier and lighter skinned Mexican citizens were routinely saved the humiliation and health risk and were allowed to cross without passing through the disinfection stations (McKiernan-González 2012). As Heide Castañeda (2019) shows, having a lighter skin tone, speaking English without an accent, and displaying markers of a higher social status continue to serve as a "phenotypic passport" that results in fewer challenges to a person's mobility across the border and within a militarized border region.

Reproduction as a Site of Racialization

Draconian immigration policies have often relied on discourses of Mexican-origin women as hyperfertile and a threat to white nationhood (Gutiérrez 2008). Mass shooters who have targeted Black and Latino people have repeated these discourses in their manifestos and online posts. A fixation on fertility reflects one of the ways through which pregnancy is a key site for understanding the reproduction of racism that drives not only anti-immigrant sentiment but also efforts of controlling the reproductive lives of Brown and Black women (Bridges 2011).

Publicly funded prenatal care in particular involves racializing practices that are contradictory in nature. While public programs for prenatal care may involve services aimed at ameliorating health inequities, there is always structural racism embedded in health institutions, health care bureaucracy, and individual-level interactions between patients and providers (Bridges 2011). The result is what Dána-Ain Davis (2019) calls obstetric racism, contributing to persistent racial disparities in birth outcomes. The biomedical realm often frames these disparities in relation to medicalized definitions of risk that draw on cultural difference to explain differential health outcomes, although "culture" may serve as a code for race, ethnicity, and class. Reproductive health care may then come with further regulation of the poor and racial minorities who accept publicly funded prenatal care alongside the increased surveillance of their "risky" bodies (Bridges 2011; Gálvez 2019; Martínez 2018).

The historical legacy of eugenics also continues to be felt by minority women. Throughout the twentieth century, poor and minority women have been forcibly sterilized (Goodwin 2020; Gutiérrez 2008; Roberts 1997) and abused as experimental subjects in the development of birth control (Ramírez de Arellano and Seipp 2017). As historian Lina-Maria Murillo (2016) documents, the Texas-Mexico border was an important region for birth control experimentation. This was largely because the maintenance of a working-class workforce to support the economy was dependent on Mexican labor, so the goal became to control the number of births, rather than eliminating the ability to reproduce. This legacy has fueled mistrust in health care institutions and providers (Rosenthal and Lobel 2020).

Eugenics influenced the medical practices and circumstances in which Mexican women in the border region gave birth throughout the early twentieth century. As Anglo doctors viewed the Mexican body as more fit for the "primitive" act of giving birth, white hospitals often denied entry of Mexican women. When admitted to hospitals, instead of birthing in the maternity wards with white women, hospital personnel instead often forced Mexicans in labor to birth alongside patients with contagious illnesses. Health officials failed to consider the high maternal and infant mortality rates among Mexicans and Mexican Americans during this period in relation to these structural inequities and racism and instead explained them away as the consequence of a culture with an unsanitary lifestyle (Sinclair 2016).

Transborder Life

To understand how immigration and border policies have widespread ramifications throughout border communities, it is necessary to understand how the US-Mexico border artificially divides places that are intimately connected. These cross-border connections fundamentally shape people's sense of identity. I often begin interviews by asking people to tell me a little bit about themselves. Lina began her response to this question by telling me where she is from: "I would say I'm from the borderland because I was born in El Paso, I was raised in Juárez, but my whole family was always in El Paso. I came to school in El Paso while living in Juárez. So it was, you know, crossing every day. Back in 2008, when I graduated high school, that's when we came and stayed [in El Paso] because of the violence [in Juárez]."

Scholars use the terms transborder and *transfronterizo* to describe the phenomenon of regularly crossing borders and how being of two places shapes experiences and identity formation in the ways Lina described (Fuentes and Peña 2010; Stephen 2007; Vélez-Ibáñez and Heyman 2017). These transborder practices reflect everyday realities of the border region, but those unfamiliar with the region often poorly understand cross-border connections. In Lina's case, her parents were Mexican citizens who crossed the border for her birth. Given that the US Constitution recognizes birthright citizenship, any baby born in the United States is a US citizen, regardless of the nationality or citizenship status of the parents. Crossing the US border with a valid visa to seek health services is within the legal rights of foreign nationals, if they provide documentation that they have paid for medical services in full. US hospitals often cater to this practice, as patients paying in full generates profit.[5] In part a result of cross-border births, there are nearly two million US citizens residing in Mexico (US Department of State 2022).

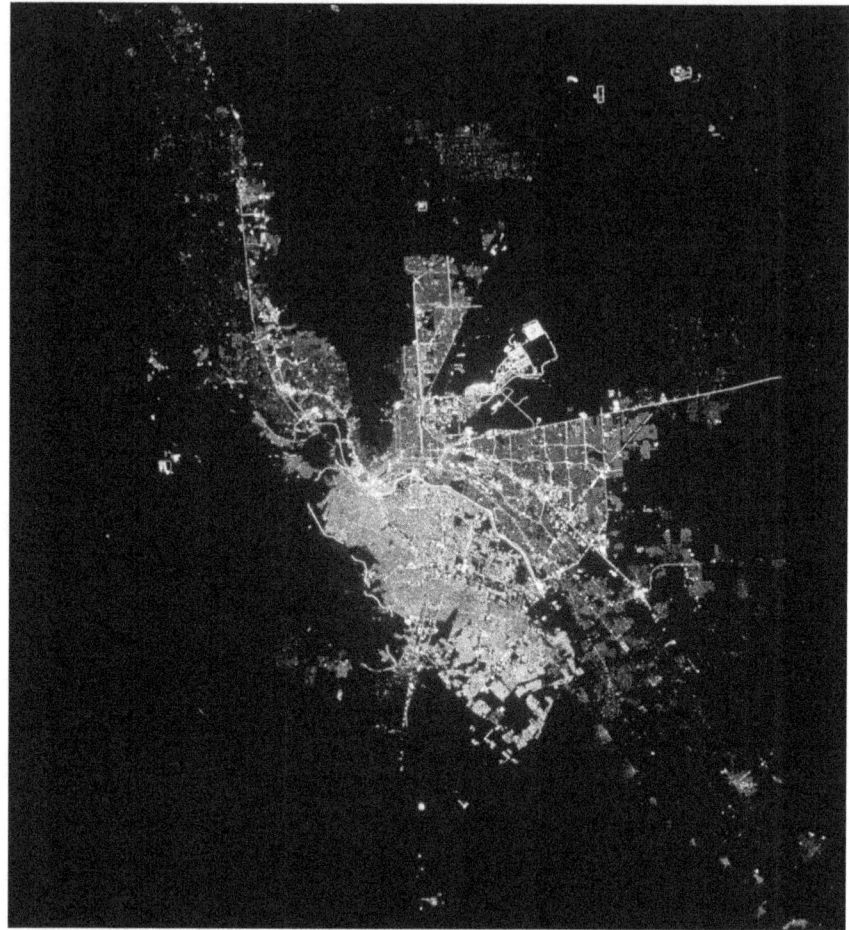

Figure I.2: The El Paso-Juárez Borderplex from space
Credit: The European Space Agency

Figure I.2 shows the sister cities from space at night. The image demonstrates how the cities exist geographically as the same urban sprawl. The international boundary is visible as a denser line, given the lighting along the border. Lina's dual citizenship facilitated her ability to live across this division. While she grew up primarily in Juárez, she crossed to El Paso daily for school, reflecting another common trend. In 2015, approximately forty thousand students regularly crossed from Mexico to the United States for school. Most of these children resided in either

Juárez or Tijuana (Orraca, Rocha, and Vargas 2017). Lina's citizenship status also eventually offered protection for her entire family. When she was finishing high school, violence was escalating in Juárez. Given her father owned a business, her family was at heightened risk of extortion and narcoviolence at the hands of warring cartels fighting over control of drug trafficking routes into the United States (Campbell 2010; Morales, Prieto, and Bejarano 2014). El Paso offered a safe haven. Her parents initially relocated without residency documents, but upon turning twenty-one, Lina legally used her citizenship status to sponsor their applications for permanent residency. While Lina's transborder life is common to the region, such practices have the potential to reinforce the border region's symbolism as a land of perpetual foreignness in the national imaginary. Lina's life trajectory, characterized by mobility across the border, also forces attention to the varied experiences of people within the border region (Heyman 2023). Lina's mobility contrasts with Brisa's vulnerability and sense of entrapment based on her immigration status. Thus, the border region is a particularly important place for questioning what epidemiologists dub the Latina Health Paradox.

Revisiting the Latina Health Paradox

Over the past several decades, there has been growing attention to the ways racism and structural vulnerabilities contribute to a higher prevalence of adverse birth outcomes among African Americans (Davis 2019; Geronimus 1992; Mullings and Wali 2001). There has been less research on adverse birth outcomes among Latinas, in part because the key birth outcomes that are most well documented—maternal deaths, infant deaths, low birth weight, and preterm birth—remain comparatively low, especially among foreign-born Latinas. Scholars have described this phenomenon as the Hispanic or Latina Health Paradox; however, a growing body of evidence suggests that researchers often fail to consider how a range of variables, such as national origin and documentation status, may factor into birth outcomes (for a review, see Montoya-Williams et al. 2021).

This lack of attention to complexity may mask other disturbing trends. Significantly, there is evidence that the Latina Health Paradox falls apart under conditions of draconian immigration enforcement

(Krieger et al. 2018; Lopez et al. 2017; Novak, Geronimus, and Martinez-Cardoso 2017), which includes a racialized deportation project that targets Latinos (Golash-Boza and Hondagneu-Sotelo 2013). Notably, there is evidence of higher burdens of mental health morbidity among Latinos within contexts of more restrictive immigration policies (Hatzenbuehler et al. 2017; Philbin et al. 2017). These emotional reactions can contribute to physiological responses tied to maternal and birth outcomes. A number of recent studies illuminate the importance of considering the association between immigration policies and birth outcomes. Importantly, Nicole Novak and colleagues (2017) found a significant increase in the prevalence of low birth weight among infants born to Latinas in Pottsville, Iowa, following a large-scale workplace immigration raid, while Krieger and colleagues (2018) found a higher incidence of preterm birth among infants born to immigrant mothers from Mexico and Central America following the 2016 election. Carmen Gutierrez and Nathan Dollar (2023) emphasize the importance of attending to nationality and temporality. They found that during the years that Trump was in office as president, infants born to both US-born and foreign-born Latinas had higher rates of preterm birth and low birth weight than infants born to these populations prior to Trump taking office. Among infants born to foreign-born women, there were significantly higher risks for those born to Mexicans and Central Americans in comparison to Puerto Ricans, Cubans, and South Americans. It is not just national-level policies that contribute to adverse outcomes. Florencia Torche and Catherine Sirois (2019) found that the passage of Arizona's SB-1070, widely viewed as anti-immigrant and promoting racial profiling, was associated with lower birthweight among infants born to Latinas in Arizona. This trend persisted, despite the lack of enforcement behind SB-1070. Further, there are variables related to maternal well-being that have been underexplored. In our own research, we found strikingly high rates of preeclampsia and gestational diabetes. Among the participants for whom we had access to medical records in our 2020–22 study, 24.9 percent had a diagnosis of preeclampsia, in comparison to a national prevalence rate of 4 percent (Bibbins-Domingo et al. 2017). The prevalence rate of gestational diabetes among participants was nearly the same, 24.7 percent, compared to a national prevalence rate of 8.3 percent (CDC 2023).

Such findings suggest a need to consider a complex range of variables, such as one's immigration status and how it has changed over time, their nationality, and their strengths of ties to the United States, as well as the immigration status of family members, when analyzing maternal health disparities. Further, there is a need to attend to what is happening in a particular place during a given period and how these contextual factors may contribute to maternal harm and adverse birth outcomes. In the border region, the enactment of immigration policies, the unfolding of the pandemic, and the aftermath of a mass shooting are all significant temporal dimensions for understanding the production of maternal harm.

August 3, 2019

On the morning of August 3, 2019, Isabela stayed at home with her three-day-old baby and toddler while her husband left to buy groceries at the Cielo Vista Walmart in central El Paso. Shortly after her husband's departure, Isabela received an active shooter emergency text alert and watched the news as reports came in on a mass shooting. The shooting left twenty-three people dead, making it one of the deadliest mass shootings and the deadliest attack on Latinos in US history. The subsequent investigation would reveal that the terrorist drove over six hundred miles to target people who looked Mexican as a response to the "Hispanic invasion of Texas," as he described in his manifesto. Revealing of the racist motivations of the attack is the fact that witnesses later reported seeing the terrorist allowing white and Black people to exit the building (see Rosas 2023). As Isabela watched the terror unfold, she tried desperately to establish contact with her husband. The cell phone towers in the area were so overwhelmed that her calls would not connect and messages would not send. It was two hours before she was able to speak with him. Fortunately, he never made it to Walmart, and instead, was trapped in the traffic created by the chaos.

Some people may view the white nationalist who murdered twenty-three people and terrorized a community as a lone wolf, given that he planned the attack and acted alone. However, sociologist Cristina Morales makes a compelling argument that the El Paso shooting should be viewed as a form of state-sponsored violence.[6] Morales's claim rests on a broader body of evidence that shows how the symbolic othering of the borderlands by those in power casts the predominately Latino population of the region as disposable, subjecting border communities to myriad forms of violence. The mass shooting was just one manifestation of state-sponsored violence in a region that has long been subjected to racially motivated attacks. Similarly, Gilberto Rosas (2023) points to the border as a place where a history of settler violence merges with the contemporary violence of immigration policy, perpetuating a mentality that incites other acts of violence such as the mass shooting. This historical legacy of violence, and how it overlaps with state-sponsored attacks on Brown bodies, includes the origins of the Texas Rangers. The Texas Rangers started out as a loosely organized militia, hired out by white settlers to carry out violence against Mexican Americans and Native Americans. The 1918 Porvenir Massacre, led by Texas Rangers who were accompanied by US soldiers, resulted in the murder of fifteen unarmed Mexicans and Mexican Americans. The attack was just one of the many racially driven acts of police, military, and Border Patrol violence against Brown bodies documented in the nineteenth and twentieth centuries (Muñoz Martinez 2018). More recently, state-sponsored border militarization has contributed to other acts of direct violence, such as migrants' deaths at the hands of immigration officials (Tahir 2019), cross-border shootings in which US Border Patrol agents have murdered people on Mexican and US soil (Morales 2019), and immigration policies that drive migrants into extreme conditions in ways that put their lives at risk (De León 2015; Rosas 2006).

While the El Paso shooter may have acted alone, without direct support of those in power, his manifesto drew inspiration from the political rhetoric of Trump, showing the ways political discourse can fuel direct violence (Piñeda 2022). Trump not only described Mexican immigrants as "rapists" and "drug dealers" while on the campaign trail, he also denigrated entire communities like El Paso that are known for being welcoming to immigrants. As Richard Piñeda points out, Trump's demonization of undocumented immigrants has the effect of demonizing broader groups of people and places perceived of as being darker or more foreign. Although the El Paso shooter reportedly aimed his WASR-10 assault rifle at Brown people, he did not make a distinction between immigrant and nonimmigrant, killing white US citizens, US citizens and residents of Mexican origin, Mexican nationals, and one German national. It was the perception of the border city as a place of foreignness that made El Paso the shooter's target.

After the massacre, Isabela said, "Now, I don't feel safe anywhere." Over a year later, a primary care physician diagnosed her with anxiety. Her experience reflects the diffuse and long-lasting effects of a mass shooting and the toll of gun violence on one's mental health. The fear of another tragedy disrupted Isabela's sense of familial security. For some, such fears overlap with other feelings of insecurity about leaving the home due to a precarious immigration status and the risk of everyday encounters with law enforcement and immigration officials. Isabela's lingering emotional trauma after the shooting is one of the many ways that mass shootings leave a lasting mark on communities. Had Isabela been pregnant at the time of the shooting, she would have been significantly more likely to experience an adverse birth outcome. Bahadir Dursun (2019) found that within a community where a mass shooting has occurred, people who are pregnant at the time of the event are significantly more likely to experience preterm delivery or give birth to a very low birthweight baby. Dursun argues this trend represents a form of intergenerational trauma, given the lifelong health implications of low birthweight and preterm birth.

The mass shooting also shows the deep connections between El Paso and Juárez. The terrorist carried out the attack on a Saturday. Weekends in the border region involve large numbers of people crossing over in both directions. On Saturdays, El Paso shopping centers are typically filled with people who reside primarily in Mexico who cross to shop, among other leisure activities. Among those who were killed and injured were people who had simply crossed over for the day to go shopping. Following the massacre, people on both sides of the border mourned and lined up to donate blood. The makeshift memorial that appeared outside of the Walmart contained flags from both countries.

The COVID-19 Pandemic in the Borderlands

While El Paso was still mourning the mass shooting, it became an epicenter of the COVID-19 pandemic. According to *El Paso Matters*, the COVID-19 death toll in Texas-Mexico border communities was "unconscionably high." Until the vaccine became widely available, the death rate for COVID-infected people under age sixty-five residing in Texas border counties was three times the national average (Kladzyk, Galewitz, and Lucas 2021). This epidemiological pattern follows a broader trend of higher risk of severe infection and death from COVID-19 among people of color (Chen and Krieger 2021). During the fall 2020 peak of the pandemic, the El Paso Convention Center served as a field hospital, and the county hospital had ten mobile morgues to store bodies. These deaths reverberated throughout the community. According to our survey data, 26 percent of participants experienced the loss of a close family member or friend due to COVID-19. This figure likely underrepresents the full death toll experienced by our participants given that we began surveys in September 2020, prior to the fall and winter peak when El Paso became one of the hardest hit cities in the United States. In part because of the severe toll of COVID-19 in El Paso, there was also widespread and relatively quick vaccine uptake. El Paso became one of the first cities in the US to fully vaccinate 70 percent of its adult population.[7]

Further exacerbating the social and economic devastation caused by the pandemic in binational communities, the Trump administration used the pandemic as a pretext to further restrict immigration and border crossing. Immigration court hearings were suspended in the early months of the pandemic. The policy known as Title 42 halted any path for asylum in the United States. All types of visa processing paused, which delayed applications for residency and naturalization. In March 2020, the United States closed its land borders to nonessential travel. This restriction lasted until November 2021, even though evidence suggests the closure had little public health benefit and incurred significant social and economic costs to border residents and asylum seekers (Maldonado 2022; Sherman-Stokes 2021). The effects of the border closure were far-reaching in communities where people are accustomed to crossing from both sides regularly for work, school, shopping, leisure, business, and visiting family. Among people we interviewed, many experienced fractured familial ties from the closure in ways that affected their well-being. These effects went beyond border communities themselves; Sarah Horton (2022) shows that Mexican immigrants in other regions of the United States were cut off from their family members, especially elders in Mexico. Immigrants and those with immigrant family members also experienced exacerbated vulnerability to the economic hardships produced by the pandemic. Some of the sectors hardest hit by the pandemic, such as the service industry, have a substantial immigrant workforce that lost employment and income, yet the Coronavirus Aid, Relief, and Economic Security (CARES) Act[8] excluded undocumented workers.

The pandemic led to a dependence on the labor of parents, especially mothers, to serve as a social safety net as the world went into lockdown. Feminist scholars of color have long commented on the ways social policies have always failed families of color (Crenshaw 1990; Davis 1983; Mullings and Wali 2001). The pandemic amplified these preexisting social inequities, creating widespread, pervasive hardships for women of color as they sought to care for their families (Eichner 2022). Ayo Wahlberg and colleagues (2021) use the term *stratified livability* to emphasize the unevenness of pandemic challenges.

The pandemic was also used as a pretext for restricting reproductive options in line with conservative political agendas. During the earliest months of the pandemic, health providers throughout the country postponed procedures defined as elective or not medically necessary. On March 22, 2020, Texas governor Greg Abbott issued an executive order to halt all nonessential health care. A press release issued the next day explicitly stated that abortions were nonessential unless the pregnant person's life was at risk. Noncompliance with the order could result in a fine or jail time. A series of appeals over the next month led the state to abandon this order, allowing abortion care to resume. However, near the beginning of the pandemic, El Paso's only abortion provider became severely ill with COVID-19. For nearly a year, El Paso was the largest US city without an abortion provider, although the geographic proximity to abortion services in New Mexico helped mitigate this lack of access to care. However, the abortion clinics in New Mexico at the time were in areas that either regularly have a substantial Border Patrol presence or required travel through an internal Border Patrol checkpoint, further exacerbating anxiety and limiting access to services for people with immigration concerns. In September 2021, Texas went on to enact one of the most restrictive abortion laws in the country, nearly eliminating access to an abortion, prior to the Supreme Court's overturn of *Roe v.*

Wade in June 2022. Texas quickly became one of fourteen states with a near total ban on abortion, and additional states may follow.

Embodiment and Local Biologies

Theoretically, the concepts of embodiment and local biologies drive this book's analysis of how the sociopolitical context of the border region translates into bodily harm. In a broad sense, embodiment refers to the ways social processes become incorporated into bodily experience (Csordas 1993; Gravlee 2009; Krieger 2016; Willen 2007). Distinct disciplinary traditions have slightly different ways of understanding embodiment as a social process. Studies of stress physiology have been important within social epidemiology, as the stress response stimulates physiological changes that increase an individual's vulnerability to a range of adverse health conditions (Krieger and Davey Smith 2004). Within anthropology, the study of embodiment has concentrated on phenomenological, lived experience (Desjarlais and Throop 2011). Phenomenological approaches emphasize the ways one's positionality and social surroundings shape how individuals engage bodily with the world, or what Thomas Csordas (1993) calls "somatic modes of attention." Sarah Willen (2007) elaborates on how somatic modes of attention relate to immigration policies, describing bodily comportment and hypervigilance during a mass deportation campaign. The altered subjectivity generated by being undocumented can also shape micropractices; actions viewed as willful behavior, such as avoiding health services, are often the consequence of constraints tied to one's immigration status (Quesada 2011).

The concept of local biologies (Lock 1993) elucidates the temporal and contextual nature of embodied vulnerabilities on the Texas-Mexico border. Local biologies attends to the entanglement of social and biological processes (Lock 2017). The characteristics of a given place at a particular moment—an unfolding pandemic, a legacy of historical injustices, limited access to health care, and the execution of policies, among other social forces—can produce biological differences but can also shape the social experience of a condition (Brotherton and Nguyen 2013; Cartwright 2011; Horton and Barker 2016; Moran-Thomas 2019). These local factors may produce disparities at the population level.

While the particularities of a place at a given moment are a key concern, this context may carry different meanings and set the stage for different embodied experiences for a person based on their social position and other individual-level factors (Nading 2017).

A focus on emotions that links embodiment and local biologies is one means for understanding how the social world translates into ill health. Emotional experiences are relational and are produced in response to the particularities of a given time and place. Those with shared geographical, historical, and social experiences may exhibit some commonalities in their vulnerabilities to particular forms of harm. Similar positionalities may condition the experiences of those harms. Emotions are also important for understanding embodiment on both the experiential and physiological levels. Emotions trigger psychological and physiological responses that can increase vulnerability to a range of ailments throughout one's life course. At the physiological level, maternal stress during pregnancy can contribute to vulnerability to adverse maternal and infant health outcomes through multiple physiological mechanisms. For example, the stress response involves the release of epinephrine and glucose. Persistent surges in epinephrine can damage arteries, increasing risk for hypertensive conditions, including preeclampsia (Wulsin et al. 2015). Consistently elevated glucose can increase vulnerability to gestational diabetes, which is associated with higher risk for preeclampsia and preterm birth (Ovesen et al. 2015). Further, epigenetic research shows how social and environmental stressors can contribute to changes in maternal gene expression; these changes are heritable and can affect the offspring (Meloni 2015). Even if changes in gene expression do not occur, environmental factors during intrauterine development can have lifelong consequences. For example, a pregnant person's burden of stress has an association with low birth weight; low birth weight is then a predictor of cardiovascular disease later in life (Kuzawa and Sweet 2009). At the experiential level, women at times linked their emotions to their bodily physiology. More often, they held explanatory models that revealed experiential forms of knowledge that stressful conditions they faced were at least in part to blame for adverse health outcomes.

Returning to Brisa, her narrative reflects a common understanding among our interlocutors of how adverse social experiences manifest as bodily harm. Brisa continually referenced feeling *presión* when seeing the border wall and immigration officials. She described the *presión* as particularly bad in the final weeks of pregnancy. *Presión* carries multiple meanings. It is often used to describe social pressures and tensions while also used colloquially to refer to high blood pressure. Brisa's narrative shows the interrelationship of these two meanings—her social world was her physiology. The constant reminders of her deportability generated a mental state of anxiety, which she associated with physiological responses in her body. Her high blood pressure was a classic symptom of preeclampsia. While preeclampsia has a complex etiology, there is substantial evidence that it is stress sensitive (Takiuti, Kahhale, and Zugaib 2003). Thus, Brisa's explanatory model and the medical literature share similar conclusions.

The relationship between maternal stress and birth outcomes is well documented. This book brings attention to women's subjective experiences to show how the social context translates into health vulnerability. The emotions women experience in response to their social world, and their perceptions of how these emotions produce health vulnerabilities, can show how policies are contributing to adverse outcomes during pregnancy, birth, and the postpartum period.

Policy Failures as Reproductive Violence

In explaining how policies contribute to harm during pregnancy, birth, and the postpartum period, I use the term *reproductive violence*. Rachelle Chadwick and Jabulile Mary-Jane Jace Mavuso (2021, 3) describe reproductive violence as the "practices, representations, policy, state, and institutional efforts to coerce, control, punish, diminish, devalue, or oppress the reproductive capacities/bodies of marginalized people." Some manifestations of reproductive violence include blatant violations of reproductive rights, such as forced sterilization and forced pregnancy. Yet, as I show in this book, reproductive violence often occurs in latent ways, relying on symbolic and structural violence to naturalize reproductive oppression.

Significant to this book is how legal violence and bureaucratic violence disenfranchise people from the health care system, even when they have legal rights to access this system. Legal violence elucidates how formally sanctioned practices have injurious effects on the lives of immigrants and their family members (Menjívar and Abrego 2012). Immigrant mothers in particular experience legal obstacles to parenting in the ways they desire (Abrego and Menjívar 2011). As previously discussed, when it comes to accessing health care, federal policies legally limit access to coverage for some categories of immigrants. This exclusion coupled with exposure to conditions that produce ill health emphasize the injurious effects of legal sanctions (Gómez Cervantes and Menjívar 2020). Although there are provisions that expand access to care during pregnancy, the bureaucratic procedures involved in utilizing publicly funded care continue to limit access to services, especially for women who are precariously documented or have mixed-status households (Heckert 2020). In effect, immigration and health policies rely on legal and bureaucratic measures that result in reproductive violence.

The effects of legal and bureaucratic violence may be uneven across place and time. Leisy Abrego and Leah Schmalzbauer (2018) argue that local factors, such as a militarized border context, create place-specific forms of legal violence. Executive orders issued under the Trump administration served to exacerbate this preexisting violence. For example, executive orders issued in 2017 expanded the criminalization of immigrants, allowing for the deportation of suspects of a crime prior to a trial or conviction (Alvord, Menjívar, and Gómez Cervantes 2018). While this legal violence arguably eased following the 2020 election, it remains clear that future changes to the law and bureaucratic procedures can contribute to widespread harm in ways that may manifest as reproductive violence.

One form of reproductive violence that has received significant scholarly attention is obstetric violence. Obstetric violence is most often described as abuse, mistreatment, dehumanized care, or neglect of patients seeking reproductive care (Castro and Savage 2019) that is a consequence of a patriarchal system aimed at controlling female and gender diverse bodies (Calvo Aguilar, Torres Falcón, and Valdez Santiago 2020). The term originated in Latin American legal frameworks. In 2007, Venezuela became the first country to grant legal recognition to the harms generated by obstetric violence, done so as a part of a law on gender-based violence (Pérez D'Gregorio 2010). Several other Latin American countries followed suit. Within the United States, obstetric violence is hypothetically encompassed under tort law, yet people's birth experiences show that even under circumstances of grievous harm, remediation through existing legal frameworks often remains out of reach (Diaz-Tello 2016). Further, legal frameworks provide recourse only when harm can be attributed to individual actors, failing to account for the structural dimensions of obstetric violence. Structural inequities contribute to obstetric violence as conditions of scarcity can lead to inadequate healthcare infrastructures that result in suboptimal care (Castro and Savage 2019; Strong 2020) and broader social inequities normalize the mistreatment of patients, especially from subaltern social groups (Castro 2019; Castro and Erviti 2014; Dixon 2015; Heckert 2016). Women of color in the United States have historically been disproportionately subjected to obstetric violence as unwilling participants in obstetric experimentation (Cooper Owens 2017; Washington 2006), the development of birth control (Ramírez de Arellano and Seipp 2017), and coerced and forced sterilization (Goodwin 2020; Gutiérrez 2008; Roberts 1997).

Often, reproductive harm occurs in covert ways. Dána-Ain Davis (2019) shows how pervasive experiences of medical racism contribute to adverse maternal and infant health outcomes among African Americans. Davis uses obstetric racism as an alternative to obstetric violence, viewing obstetric violence as inadequate for capturing the role of race in obstetric encounters. Further, structural racism exacerbates the effects of obstetric violence to fuel a disproportionate burden of adverse birth outcomes among people of African descent in the United States and other places where Black people are a racialized minority (Davis 2019; Williamson 2021). Other racialized groups experience similar patterns of obstetric racism. In Mexico, those perceived of as more Indigenous because of poverty, low educational attainment, or being from a rural area, often experience mistreatment at the hands of providers. Abuses include the overuse of interventions that result in iatrogenic harm. Justifications for unnecessary interventions are often related to perceptions that those from marginalized backgrounds are more likely to have riskier births, showing the harms that arise from racializing risk (Dixon 2015; Smith-Oka 2022). This important scholarship shows how structural violence, and especially structural racism, are fundamental not only to obstetric violence but also to other experiences of reproductive harm that occur beyond the clinical context.

The experiences of Brisa and others highlight that focusing only on obstetric violence is insufficient for understanding the production of maternal harm. In Brisa's case, her experiences of reproductive violence went beyond the clinical context. In fact, she described a positive birth experience where she felt respected and well cared for by her Certified Nurse Midwife (CNM), whom she referred to as a doctor, and nurses. She said, "The people who attended the birth were very good, even the doctor. I liked my birth. I was aware of what was happening and I could touch the baby's head before she was completely out. It felt very harmonious." As we will see, many research participants used midwives or OB-GYNs (doctors of obstetrics and gynecology) within a practice that had a strong midwifery presence. This detail may have allowed for more positive clinical encounters given that midwifery involves practices aimed at respecting the dignity and social well-being of the birthing person (Rooks 1999). For Brisa, harm came not from her care, but through her embodied experience of immigration policies that caused her to live in a constant state of anxiety and health policies that limited her access to optimal care. Other interlocutors described experiences of obstetric violence as it related to mistreatment and neglect by their providers, and it remains important to understand these experiences in relation to social inequities and health policies. My use of the term reproductive violence facilitates a focus on how the structural dimensions produced via immigration, health, and social policies manifest as maternal harm. The clinical context accounts for only some dimensions of this harm.

Attending to the production of reproductive violence beyond the clinical realm draws inspiration from reproductive justice. Ciara Laverty and Dieneke de Vos (2021) describe reproductive violence as including "violations of reproductive autonomy and self-determination: the ability to decide if, when, how, and under what conditions to have and raise children" (112). This framing creates a direct contrast to reproductive justice, which advocates for the right to have (or not have) a child in conditions of dignity, while considering the variables of oppression that constrain individual choice. Reproductive justice politicizes reproductive rights by centering race, class, gender, immigration status, and other axes of marginalization. It considers the structural, legal, and interpersonal dynamics that limit reproductive autonomy, generate maternal harm, and limit the ability of individuals to make decisions about family rearing under dignified conditions (Hernandez and De Los Santos Upton 2019; Roberts 2015; Ross 2017; Valdez and Deomampo 2019; Zavella 2020). Reproductive justice encourages a focus beyond the clinical experience to consider the ways in which racism, socioeconomic inequities, immigration policy, and other variables of oppression lead to harm during the course of reproductive life events. The goals of reproductive justice suggest a need to consider the scope, temporality, and individual positionality within broader power arrangements as they relate to the experience of reproduction.

The term reproductive injustice has been more commonly used to draw contrasts to reproductive justice (see Davis 2019; Lira and Stern 2014; Messing, Fabi, and Rosen 2020) and to describe patterns that I am attributing to reproductive violence. While reproductive injustice captures much of what I have described in defining reproductive violence, I opt to use terminology that includes violence to emphasize the harm that is a direct consequence of social injustices. In essence, reproductive violence is about the various forms of structural, symbolic, and legal violence that coalesce to cause maternal harm. Much of this harm is normalized and remains invisible, as it fails to register in the clinical realm, except when it manifests as a severe adverse birth outcome. In line with Chadwick and Jace Mavuso (2021), I view the term reproductive violence as an effort to challenge the social conditions that produce patterns of harm and demand better conditions for parents as they reproduce, give birth, and care for their children.

Researching Maternal Health and Emotional Distress

Two related studies on maternal health and emotional distress inform this book. As noted earlier, I led the first study from 2018 to 2019 and the second from 2020 to 2022. These different periods capture distinct landscapes in relation to the enactment of immigration policy and the unfolding of the COVID-19 pandemic. Taken together, they demonstrate that even as events unfold and policies shift, the long-standing patterns that contribute to health disparities in the region persist.

From 2018 to 2019, I focused on how immigration-related concerns shaped the emotional experience of pregnancy. This coincided with a period of heightened anxiety over seeking health care as a consequence of threats of immigration enforcement under the Trump administration (Callaghan et al. 2019). To capture the effects of immigration policies, we interviewed twenty-five first-generation immigrants and ten second-generation immigrants, meaning at least one parent was born outside of the United States. Of the foreign-born participants, all but three were born in Mexico. One was born in Venezuela and, since we did not limit the focus to Latina immigrants for this study, the other two were born in Kenya and the Gambia, respectively. We recruited participants by working with community organizations that provide support for pregnant and postpartum individuals, including community clinics and food pantries. From 2020 to 2022, my research moved into a clinical context and involved 176 participants who were seeking prenatal care through the county's public safety-net hospital and its associated OB-GYN and midwifery practice. All interlocutors in this study were utilizing either CHIP Perinatal or Medicaid for Pregnant Women, except for one who was classified as self-pay. This project also included the collection of survey data, cortisol samples, and medical records. In this book, I draw primarily from the interviews we conducted with a subsample of women, although there are places where I reference statistics from the larger study. Appendix I provides a discussion of our methods for integrating cortisol samples into anthropological work. Most of the initial interviews we conducted with sixty participants took place while the person was still pregnant, although some took place postpartum. Fourteen of these individuals participated in additional interviews during the first year postpartum. Of the interview participants, eighteen were born in Mexico and one was born in Chile but had grown up in Mexico before immigrating to the United States. The remaining forty-one women were US-born citizens, seven of whom had spent at least significant portions of their childhood in Mexico. While a majority of women were US-born citizens, their narratives often captured the ways immigration policies infiltrated their lives via their connections to others and residence on the border. Of the US-born citizens, twenty-four were second-generation immigrants and thirteen described having immigration-related concerns for immediate family members or intimate partners. Appendix II provides a summary of participants from both projects. We complemented both studies with additional interviews with providers, employees of community and social service organizations, and policymakers.

From 2018 to 2019, interviews took place in person in a mutually agreed upon location, which was most often the participant's home. From 2020 to 2022, the public health threat of the pandemic required that we begin the project using virtual methods, which included phone and Zoom interviews. During the summer of 2021, we began offering the option of meeting in person for interviews, but we quickly switched back to virtual methods with the emergence of the Delta and Omicron variants. The heightened risk for pregnant people and newborns came with an ethical imperative to continue with extra precautions, even as people began navigating a new normal. Conducting interviews virtually entails challenges as well as advantages. I often felt like I was missing some of the ethnographic details that emerge through in-person encounters—reading body language, having interruptions and interactions with family members, and seeing the context of people's lives within their homes. Some people even stated that there were things that would be easier to explain in person. Conversely, other interlocutors said that the increased anonymity of a phone interview made it easier for them to talk about difficult issues. Additionally, individuals who may have been less likely to participate due to time constraints, which is often the case for new parents, found it easier to arrange a virtual interview. Overall, the 2020–22 project involved an adaptation of methodologies in response to the constraints of the pandemic.

Although writing this book has been a sole endeavor, the research behind it was a collaborative effort. From 2018 to 2019, several undergraduate students helped with conducting, transcribing, and analyzing interviews. The 2020–22 project involved an interdisciplinary team of researchers that included a sociologist, two neuroscientists, a public health expert, an OB-GYN, and several medical students. These colleagues have been instrumental in conducting provider interviews as well as the analysis of quantitative data, health records, and cortisol samples that were a part of this project. Again, I was fortunate to mentor a number of graduate and undergraduate students who assisted with data collection and analysis. In both projects, I conducted roughly half of the interviews, while students conducted the other half. At times, the insights from these students have influenced my own analysis as presented in this book. Many of these students have taken authorship roles in other pieces produced from our research (see De Anda and Heckert

2022; Heckert and Mata under review; Maldonado 2022; Solis and Heckert 2021). Throughout this book, I often use "we" to acknowledge the collaborative efforts of the data collection process.

During the course of this research, I became pregnant and became a parent. My own vantage point is one of privilege, as I am white, married, highly educated, and financially stable. However, the challenges I experienced from the timing of my pregnancy and birth mirrored some of those experienced by my interlocutors, although in many cases I had access to resources that mitigated the effects of these crises. When the mass shooting occurred on August 3, 2019, my husband and I had recently decided we wanted to have a baby. Weeks later, I was pregnant. Fresh on my mind was the knowledge that the shooter aimed to murder people who looked like my husband, a Bolivian immigrant, and (possibly) our future child. When the initial pandemic lockdown unfolded in mid-March of 2020, I was seven months pregnant and quite anxiety-ridden over the unknown. I had already planned a home birth prior to the pandemic, and the anticipation of an overwhelmed hospital system reinforced my desire to avoid a hospital delivery. However, at thirty-eight weeks' gestation, I developed preeclampsia and my son was breech. This combination of factors required a transfer to hospital care and led to a C-section. Like many of my interlocutors, I found the postpartum period in the middle of a pandemic to be extremely isolating and lonely. Yet, the social advantages that I had gave my family a sense of security. Teaching summer school is optional at the institution where I am a professor, and I was in a position to take the summer off following a May birth, although I still ended up grading final papers from my hospital bed. My husband is a teacher and was also able to have the summer free from work obligations. Our timing gave us both three months of paid parental leave—benefits that the United States and Texas fail to provide to most parents. In comparison, nearly one in four birthing people return to work within two weeks of the birth, and this period is even shorter for the nonbirthing parent (Lerner 2015). During the pandemic, new parents had to navigate decisions about returning to work with fears that exposure within their work environments would put their newborns at risk of COVID-19. While the death rate from COVID-19 is far lower for newborns than older adults, the hospitalization rate of infants diagnosed with COVID-19 is six times higher than that of other children under the age of five (Allen et al. 2022). Additionally, the vaccine was unavailable to children under five until the summer of 2022, over a year after the vaccine became widely available to adults in the United States. Under normal circumstances, parental leave policies in the United States are failing new parents. During the pandemic, a lack of protective polices created impossible dilemmas. My own positionality, which involves having a job I could do remotely through the worst of the pandemic, protected me from having to make a decision about whether to leave a job in order to better protect and care for a newborn child at home.

Like many of my interlocutors, I have also at times had immigration-related concerns for family members. My husband came to the US with his family on a tourist visa when he was fifteen years old. It was not until we married that he was able to adjust his legal status through marriage to a US citizen. When he became a naturalized citizen, he was able to petition for residency for his parents. Prior to our marriage, we lived in an area in which the local sheriff's department had entered into a 287(g) agreement under which law enforcement officials were deputized to perform the functions of immigration officials. The result was that routine traffic stops could easily lead to deportations. For my husband, his family, and myself, there was a constant awareness of this threat to familial unity.

These details about my own experience are to illustrate how my own story informs my research and writing. In interviews and conversations, I often shared my experiences as a way to establish common ground with interlocutors, and we often talked about shared experiences and emotions. However, my position of privilege has protected me from the more severe hardships experienced by many of the people I interviewed.

Overview of Chapters

In what follows, I continue to explore the various ways policies contribute to physical and emotional harm during pregnancy, birth, and the postpartum period. Chapter 1, "Legislating Maternal Harm," further explains how the intersection of immigration and health policies stratifies access to prenatal and postpartum care and the implications of this stratification for maternal health. Chapter 2, "Immigration Policy and

Embodied Vulnerability," focuses on the role of immigration policies in producing emotional distress and how women perceived their emotions as being related to their health and the health of their babies. It includes attention to how immigration-related concerns extend beyond one's own immigration status, as women's concerns over others factored into their own sense of well-being. Chapter 3, "The Local Biology of Preeclampsia," gives attention to a specific stress-sensitive health condition, preeclampsia, which had an alarmingly high prevalence rate among our research participants. I use narratives of people diagnosed with preeclampsia to explore the role of their social experiences in producing vulnerabilities to this condition and attend to how existing health and social policies fail to address these vulnerabilities.

The second half of the book involves a greater focus on experiences during the pandemic. Chapter 4, "Conjugated Harm and Pregnancy during the Pandemic"; Chapter 5, "Finding Compassionate Care"; and Chapter 6, "Navigating *Impotencia* during the Postpartum Period," taken together, examine pregnancy, birth, and postpartum experiences during the pandemic and the role of border, public health, and social policies, combined with insufficient safety nets, in shaping these experiences. Chapter 5 includes reflections on the role of midwifery and community clinics in enabling people to find compassionate care, while considering the challenges to expanding access to these forms of care, especially for people using publicly funded prenatal care. The conclusion offers reflections on measures that could help alleviate the types of challenges faced by my interlocutors as a part of continued efforts of achieving reproductive justice.

1

Legislating Maternal Harm

Anessa: Coverage under CHIP Perinatal

In January 2022, Anessa gave birth to her first child in El Paso, Texas. Upon admission to the hospital, her and her husband tested positive for COVID-19, which came as a surprise to her. They were both vaccinated and asymptomatic, and Anessa had avoided leaving the house for two months leading up to the birth over fear of the high number of breakthrough infections with the Omicron variant. In the weeks following the birth, she developed mastitis, a bacterial infection of breast tissue. Typically caused by lactation, the symptoms of mastitis include pain, swelling, and fever. However, Anessa's condition became so severe that it required surgical drainage of multiple abscesses. The breast abscesses that she experienced are rare, usually only occurring as a complication of untreated mastitis.

The severity of Anessa's condition was in large part a consequence of the type of coverage she had. Given that she was in the process of adjusting her immigration status via marriage to a US citizen, she only qualified for Children's Health Insurance Program (CHIP) Perinatal—a program that limits coverage to conditions classified as posing a risk to the fetus. Anessa's lack of postpartum coverage, combined with her COVID-19 diagnosis, led to delays in treating her mastitis. Because she was COVID-19 positive at the time of the birth, she did not receive a visit from a lactation consultant, which she believes contributed to her lack of awareness of the earliest symptoms of the condition. She said, "I didn't know I had mastitis. I was in a lot of pain, but I thought I could tolerate it." Things quickly progressed, but she was unable to get an in-person appointment because she had not yet completed her ten-day COVID-19 isolation period. She said, "Then I had fevers and my head always hurt. My breast was always hurting and I could not carry the baby on that side. Even at WIC[1] they did not want to see me because I had COVID." When she was able to schedule a postpartum visit, her provider told her that she had postpartum depression and mastitis. The doctor gave her no referral for the former and directed her to the emergency room for the latter. Since CHIP Perinatal would not cover treatment for mastitis and her condition was not deemed life-threatening, the emergency room turned her away. She explained how the situation progressed: "When I went to my appointment, the doctor tried to help me. But it was a problem with the hospital. They did not help me or give me economic help. Or maybe they didn't grasp that I didn't have help from insurance. So, I had to find a surgeon outside of the hospital." In the emergency room, no one offered her an application for the hospital system's charity care program or a payment plan. She decided her only option was to seek care across the border in Juárez, Mexico.

Although Anessa was born and raised in Juárez, she feared trying to cross back into the US before securing her green card. She could indeed have faced significant problems. While Anessa described herself as being in the process of adjusting her status, her lawyer had not yet submitted the paperwork to United States Citizenship and Immigration Services (USCIS) to begin the review process. Since Anessa's husband did not earn enough money to be the sole sponsor of her petition, they needed a cosponsor. An aunt had agreed to cosponsor the petition, but they were having trouble collecting the required documents from her to complete the paperwork. Anessa did have an unexpired border crossing card that she obtained prior to her marriage, which she used to travel to Mexico to treat her mastitis. A border crossing card is similar to a tourist visa, but only issued to Mexican citizens for travel within the designated border zone for up to thirty days. Had it been just a few months earlier, during the extended closure of the border during the pandemic, Anessa would have been unable to enter the United States with only a border crossing card. Further, given that she had previously overstayed the thirty-day limit, hypothetically, immigration officials could have denied her reentry. Fortunately, Anessa crossed back without trouble. However, finding a provider and scheduling an appointment in Juárez led to further delays in her care. In the meantime, she had pus leaking from her breast and she ceased breastfeeding. Her dedication to providing her child breastmilk was clear, as she sought donated breastmilk from a number of friends who had a frozen surplus. Unfortunately, she was never able to reinitiate breastfeeding, making her feel like she failed her child, which exacerbated her postpartum depression.

Salma: Coverage under Medicaid for Pregnant Women

Salma is a US-born citizen who gave birth to her third child in the summer of 2021. She experienced multiple complications during the pregnancy, delivery, and postpartum period. In the year leading up to her pregnancy, she learned she had developed type 2 diabetes and expressed concern that she was unable to manage her diet and exercise in the ways that she wanted to during the pregnancy. Given her fear of contracting COVID-19 while pregnant, she was not working, which created economic hardship that impacted her family's food budget. She also described how her family members, who worked in the funeral business and were seeing many COVID-19 deaths, were so overprotective of her that she felt like she could not even go for walks outside to exercise.

Salma had a planned C-section, a decision based on her history of two previous C-sections. The procedure involved complications related to the buildup of scar tissue from the earlier surgeries. The complications led to vacuum suction to assist in the removal of the baby and resulted in significant blood loss and hours of surgery. During the procedure, Salma's legs began shaking uncontrollably, which created additional challenges and resulted in the anesthesiologist administering drugs that caused her to hallucinate. Although Salma had planned to have a tubal ligation as an add-on procedure to the C-section, given the complications, this was not possible.

Postpartum, Salma underwent a difficult recovery from the arduous surgery. She also began experiencing challenges controlling her blood sugar alongside symptoms of high blood pressure. Given she could not fathom having to undergo yet another surgery to proceed with the tubal ligation, she opted for an intrauterine device (IUD). Exacerbating her postpartum challenges was the fact that her Medicaid was set to expire—or so she thought.

The Families First Coronavirus Response Act required states to provide continuous coverage to Medicaid enrollees through the duration of the COVID-19 public health emergency declaration in order to be eligible for federal funds. Individuals enrolled in Medicaid for Pregnant Women at any time during the public health emergency should have received continuous coverage postpartum until states received authorization to begin recertifying Medicaid recipients in anticipation of the end of the public health emergency on May 11, 2023. Yet, Salma, like many of the postpartum people we interviewed who had Medicaid for Pregnant Women, gave us a specific expiration date for her coverage.

Based on interviews with social service providers as well as follow-up with people who thought their Medicaid coverage had ended or would be ending, it became clear that while Texas was not actively disenrolling people from Medicaid, bureaucratic procedures led people to believe their coverage had expired. I will delve into further details about this later in the chapter. For Salma, thinking that her coverage would expire shaped her decisions about her health and generated a fear that she would have to struggle to get the care she needed for her diabetes and blood pressure. In an interview shortly before she thought her coverage expired, Salma rattled off the measures she planned to take to find care, starting with applying to the public hospital's discount program. It was through these subsequent interactions with social service providers that she discovered she could maintain access to Medicaid. Although Texas Health and Human Services (HHS) insists that continued enrollment in Medicaid during the pandemic was an automatic process, Salma had a different understanding of events; "I had to ask for it," Salma explained.

Stratified Access to Maternal Health Care

The different landscapes of care that characterized Anessa and Salma's health experiences are in part a consequence of stratified access to prenatal care. Stratified access refers to the ways health policies and systems lead to differential access to health services. Social categorizations, including immigration status, contribute to this stratification (Castañeda 2018). Immigration status has not always factored into inclusion criteria for health programs, and health care stratification has evolved in relation to immigration and welfare policies.[2] Currently, in Texas, Medicaid and CHIP Perinatal are the safety-net programs that provide coverage for prenatal care, delivery, and, to some extent, postpartum care. As table 1.1 shows, immigration status is the primary factor that

TABLE 1.1: Comparison of Texas's Publicly Funded Prenatal Care Programs

Program	Immigration requirements	Income requirements	Coverage (During Time of Research)
Medicaid for Pregnant Women	US Citizenship or at least 5 years of legal permanent residency	198% FPL or below	Comprehensive care during pregnancy, the birth, and the 60 days postpartum
CHIP Perinatal	Evidence of living in Texas, but no exclusion based on immigration status	202% FPL or below	Prenatal appointments and coverage for conditions defined as posing a risk to the fetus Delivery, but not false labor Up to 2 postpartum visits, but no coverage for additional postpartum services

determines which program a person will gain coverage under. Given that Medicaid for Pregnant Women offers comprehensive coverage, while CHIP Perinatal coverage is much more limited, immigration status determines the standard of care a person can access.

The limited care provided through CHIP Perinatal is a reflection of political agendas aimed at denying services to immigrant populations while at the same time establishing frameworks for recognizing fetal personhood. The George W. Bush administration granted states the option to use federal funding under CHIP to provide coverage to the unborn US citizen. States have some control in determining what specific services CHIP Perinatal will cover, but they cannot use federal funds for health services not intended to benefit the child.[3] In 2007, the Texas legislature voted to utilize the CHIP Perinatal option, in large part because conservative legislators interpreted the program as granting personhood to the fetus, providing an opportunity to establish precedence for restricting abortion access (Fabi 2019). While passage of CHIP Perinatal in Texas was significant for expanding access to prenatal care, it came at the cost of undermining other dimensions of reproductive justice (Cleek 2019).[4]

The ways CHIP Perinatal provides coverage for the US-citizen fetus while ignoring the comprehensive health needs of the noncitizen mother perpetuates what Elizabeth Farfán-Santos (2019) describes as a womb-body divide. It is the womb, nurturing a future US citizen, which the law deems worthy of care, while the mother's body is undeserving of the same standard of care. The CHIP Perinatal Member Handbook published by El Paso Health, one of the managed care networks subcontracted by Medicaid and CHIP programs in Texas, contains numerous reminders that coverage is "for your unborn baby" (El Paso Health 2022). This handbook is also telling of the other contradictions inherent to prioritizing the womb. In the case of a miscarriage, CHIP Perinatal will cover the costs of follow-up care, but only if the pregnant person has already obtained coverage prior to the miscarriage. For a person who is already having a miscarriage but still pending approval from the program, CHIP Perinatal will not cover the costs of care. It reinforces the notion that the pregnant person's health only matters when it is carrying a future citizen.

How CHIP Perinatal handles miscarriage is one of many contradictions that result from covering the fetus while denying coverage for other health issues the pregnant person may have. As a Certified Nurse Midwife (CNM) explained, "The health of the mother always has implications for the fetus." From her perspective, it is unclear who gets to decide what counts as pregnancy-related services for the purpose of CHIP Perinatal coverage, as is the rationale for such decisions. For example, Texas CHIP Perinatal does not cover disease management of preexisting conditions, but thirteen states do use federal funds under CHIP to provide these services. Further, Texas and Tennessee are the only states that do not provide coverage for emergency services under CHIP Perinatal. While CHIP Perinatal in Texas clearly prioritizes the fetus over the pregnant person, to a lesser extent, Texas Medicaid also reinforces the womb-body divide. Texas is among the states with the strictest eligibility criteria for Medicaid. In 2023, a dual parent household with two children would need to earn less than $285 per month in order for the parents to qualify for coverage as the caretakers of a minor (Texas HHS 2023). However, Medicaid for Pregnant Women will cover a pregnant person who earns up to 198 percent of the federal poverty level (FPL). The much more generous income threshold for coverage during pregnancy suggests that it is only when the womb is growing a fetus that the state deems a person worthy of care under Medicaid.

Even with the limitations imposed by CHIP Perinatal, this program does offer access to care that is not available in all states. For example, neighboring New Mexico is one of twenty-nine states that has not adopted the CHIP Perinatal provision or used state funds to extend

Medicaid to undocumented pregnant people. In these states, those who do not qualify for Medicaid coverage due to immigration issues instead rely on access to prenatal care through a combination of Title X clinics,[5] local safety-net programs, and out-of-pocket payment, or they forego prenatal care and deliver under Emergency Medicaid.

Medicaid and CHIP Perinatal both offer limited postpartum care, although the limitations are greater for those utilizing CHIP Perinatal. Those covered under Medicaid for Pregnant Women are automatically enrolled in Healthy Texas Women (HTW) following the birth. HTW is limited in scope, providing annual wellness exams and contraception access. For the first twelve months postpartum, Healthy Texas Women Plus (HTW+) also provides coverage for some services necessary to manage the three most common health conditions that contribute to maternal mortality and morbidity: substance abuse, cardiovascular disease, and postpartum depression.[6] The program also has the same exclusion criteria as Medicaid programs, meaning that individuals with CHIP Perinatal most likely cannot qualify for HTW.

In light of increasing maternal mortality rates in the United States (MacDorman et al. 2016; MacDorman et al. 2018), there have been state-level efforts to implement maternal mortality task forces. Data collected by the Texas Maternal Mortality and Morbidity Task Force (Texas DSHS 2018) revealed that in Texas, 70 percent of maternal deaths that occurred between 2012 and 2015 were among individuals covered by Medicaid and 56 percent of maternal deaths occurred after the sixty-day-postpartum Medicaid cutoff. This data has helped support efforts to extend postpartum Medicaid coverage; however, there has been little effort to expand postpartum coverage under CHIP Perinatal. When the American Rescue Plan (2021) gave states the option to extend pregnancy Medicaid to twelve months postpartum, Texas HB-133 sought to use federal funding to provide this extended coverage. While the initial bill aimed to provide a full year of postpartum coverage, the state senate amended the bill to only provide coverage for six months postpartum. Under HB-133, the extended coverage would take effect on September 1, 2021. However, the Centers for Medicare and Medicaid determined the Texas law violated federal guidelines. Had the law extended coverage for a full twelve months postpartum in line with guidelines under the American Rescue Plan, Texas's plan would have been automatically approved for federal funding. Given the Texas law deviated from the federal guidelines by only proposing six months of extended coverage, the Centers for Medicare and Medicaid had to provide a full review of the proposal. Language that would deny postpartum Medicaid coverage to those with an "intended miscarriage,"[7] which includes people who had a medically necessary abortion, prevented HB-133 from receiving federal approval. As a result, when the COVID-19 public health emergency ended, postpartum coverage under Medicaid returned to ending at sixty days after the birth. Once again, during the 2023 legislative session, Texas passed a law to extend Medicaid for Pregnant Women. This time, the law would extend coverage for a full year postpartum, in accordance with federal guidelines. Yet, the law still contains language that would deny postpartum coverage to a person who has an abortion. At the time of writing, the law is pending federal approval.

There may be differential birth outcomes associated with stratified access to prenatal care, although there is minimal research on these disparities. State Medicaid programs, including CHIP programs, undergo periodic external reviews that compile data on maternal mortality, severe maternal morbidity, NICU (neonatal intensive care unit) transfers, and low birth weight. The most recent external reviews of Texas Medicaid programs suggest that severe maternal morbidity and maternal mortality are significantly lower among those with coverage under CHIP Perinatal in comparison to those with coverage under Medicaid (Texas DSHS 2019, 2020, 2021). This may be counterintuitive given that CHIP Perinatal provides less comprehensive coverage, but it aligns with what researchers have dubbed the Latina Health Paradox. This paradox describes the phenomenon that recent Latina immigrants tend to have healthier births than immigrants with longer lengths of residency and their US-born counterparts do, despite having less access to healthcare services and other structural constraints. A growing body of research suggests that this paradox is more complex than many models account for, especially when considering the diversity of nationalities, immigration statuses, and migration histories that researchers tend to lump together under the classification of Latina (Montoya-Williams et al. 2021). Critiques of the paradox arise in part from poor data collection that limits better disaggregation of data. Medical records and birth certificate data are commonly used sources of data, yet both only offer insights on a limited set of variables. The Pregnancy Risk Assessment Monitoring System (PRAMS) is another one of the most widely used sources of data on postpartum outcomes, yet this survey also leaves data gaps. In particular, the PRAMS survey questions do a poor job distinguishing between coverage under CHIP Perinatal and Medicaid, making it impossible to compare outcomes for births covered under these programs. Further, hard-to-reach groups covered under CHIP Perinatal tend to be underrepresented in such surveys. Consequently, there may be a failure to document a broader range of disparities in birth and postpartum outcomes.

The fact that it may appear that birth outcomes are better under CHIP Perinatal than Medicaid can be misconstrued to support the argument that CHIP Perinatal provides sufficient coverage. As Salma's and Anessa's experiences highlight, both CHIP Perinatal and Medicaid for Pregnant Women involve policies and legislative decisions that constrain the actions a person can take when responding to their reproductive health needs. While there may be differences in the birth outcomes based on type of coverage, women's narratives showed common patterns behind adverse outcomes with both programs. First, the bureaucratic measures involved in both programs led to different degrees of exclusion among those who qualified for coverage. Second, many women included under both programs had no insurance outside of being pregnant, and their limited and temporary inclusion in coverage was insufficient for addressing a lifetime of exclusion from health care. Finally, both programs posed significant limitations for achieving reproductive justice against a backdrop characterized by increasing restrictions on bodily autonomy. Reproductive experiences suggest that while stratified access creates different dynamics of constraints in access to care, the limitations imposed by both programs allow for adverse experiences and health outcomes.

The Bureaucratic Violence of Navigating Publicly Funded Prenatal Care

Jazmine provided exact dates of when she believed her coverage under Medicaid for Pregnant Women ended following her two pandemic births—one in June 2020 and another in March 2022. She also had a toddler, born prior to the pandemic. Given the requirements for states to maintain continuous coverage under Medicaid during the public health emergency, hypothetically, she should have continued to have Medicaid coverage between her two most recent pregnancies and well beyond our postpartum interview in June 2022. However, according to Jazmine, her coverage expired shortly after the delivery of each of her children.

Jazmine and Salma reflect a common pattern of people thinking their Medicaid coverage had expired postpartum, unaware that they were entitled to continuous coverage during the public health emergency. Of the postpartum interviews we conducted from 2020 to 2022, fifteen were with individuals who had Medicaid for Pregnant Women. Over half of those individuals initially reported that their Medicaid had expired or was set to expire, with some women providing exact expiration dates. In trying to figure out what was going on, we interviewed a low-level HHS employee who explained that following the birth, people receive renewal notices when their expiration dates come up. People are able to submit requested information on their own, but many submit it through an HHS employee either over the phone or in person. On her end, she reported struggling to make contact with people when their renewal notices came up. When people preferred to come in for an appointment to submit their information, they often had excessively long wait times due to understaffing issues. She explained further:

> When we let them know, "Hey, times up, you got to send this in," they may miss that. And then, with the one call that I try, they may miss that because they're trying to work or they're doing something with their kids. So, there's a lot of challenges. I think having that one opportunity, the one time we mail it out, the one time we give them a call, you know they may miss it all. You know there are many times where I don't get to interview somebody because they're missing the phone calls. It's more often that I'm not able to interview someone than I get a hold of somebody. And if somebody never got the information, they never got the opportunity.

This HHS employee later expressed significant distress over the process, which she also believed was leading people to lose their Medicaid coverage.

Feeling enraged by these findings, I put together a research brief that I disseminated to local legislators. The office of State Representative Lina Ortega subsequently began inquiry with Texas HHS. HHS was adamant that they had not dropped anyone from Medicaid and affirmed that renewal under the program was automatic. However, this questioning also revealed that HHS did in fact send renewal notices every six months with confusing language that included expiration dates (see figure 1.1). One participant shared a copy of this renewal notice with me. Within the thirty-six-page document, there is no mention that Medicaid recipients would receive extended coverage during the pandemic. Instead, most of the document solicits information to renew benefits, prefaced with the warning "If we don't get your renewal on time, your benefits might end." According to HHS's response to an inquiry from Representative Ortega's office, even if a beneficiary did not respond to the renewal notice, they still maintained Medicaid coverage through the duration of the public health emergency. It remains unclear why HHS sent these renewal notices in the first place, given the human resource strain and administrative costs associated with this extra paperwork. The fact that even an employee of the agency thought that failure to respond to the renewal notice led a person to lose their Medicaid shows the extent to which the paperwork misled people.

As these details unfolded, I began reaching out to people who initially reported that their Medicaid coverage had expired or who were unsure if they had maintained coverage. Fortunately, all the people I reconnected with had eventually discovered that they continued to have coverage. This may have been in part because I began prompting people to look into it when this issue came up during interviews. In some instances, people were actively seeking care or applying to other social service programs when they discovered they still had Medicaid.

While perhaps Texas HHS did not officially drop anyone from Medicaid, people's belief that they no longer had coverage caused them to operate as if they did not have insurance. Jazmine described having postpartum depression after the birth of her second child. She never received a diagnosis, however, since she felt too unwell to go to a postpartum visit prior to the expiration date of her Medicaid. Months later, she still felt like she needed support, which she never sought because of her assumption that she lacked coverage. According to Jazmine, she

> **It is time to renew your benefits.**
> The benefits you need to renew have a check-mark next to them:
>
> ☐ SNAP   ☐ TANF   ☒ Health Care
>
> **You can renew benefits online or by returning the form that came with this letter.**
> **To renew online:** Go to YourTexasBenefits.com, log in and click 'Manage'. Find the case that says 'Ready for renewal' and click 'Details'. Click 'Renew Benefits' to begin.
> **To renew using the form that came with this letter:** Return the form by mail using the pre-paid envelope or by fax. The fax number is listed above. Don't forget to sign the form.
>
> **Due dates:**
> Send your online renewal form or the form with this letter as soon as you can. If we don't get your renewal in time, your benefits might end.
>
> | Health Care (EDG ▓▓▓) | Your current health care benefits end 12/2022. |
> |---|---|
>
> Need help filling out the form? **Call 2-1-1 (toll free).**

Figure 1.1: Section from a Texas HHS benefits renewal notice sent to a Medicaid for Pregnant Women recipient (the full renewal notice is thirty-six pages)

received no information about the possibility that her coverage could be extended. She also described an unmet need for birth control between her second and third child; on the survey, she reported a lack of health coverage and lack of affordability as among the factors shaping her decisions about birth control. This unmet need ultimately contributed to an unplanned pregnancy. She had recently recovered from COVID-19 and was still breastfeeding when she became pregnant with her third child. She attributed her changes in appetite and nausea to her loss of taste and smell from COVID-19 and the continued absence of her period was nothing unexpected while breastfeeding. Consequently, she was already twenty weeks pregnant when she decided to visit a doctor in Juárez.

Jazmine described delays in having her Medicaid application processed when she applied again in the summer of 2021. After submitting her initial application, she did not receive a response and had to resubmit the application and, finally, call HHS in order to get her benefits card, which further delayed her initiation of prenatal care until she was twenty-three weeks pregnant. After the delivery in the spring of 2022, she again believed her Medicaid had expired two months postpartum. After the birth, she attempted to schedule a postpartum visit multiple times, describing a desire to take better care of herself so that she would not experience postpartum depression again. However, on the date of her postpartum visit, she lost her wallet and missed her appointment.

She was unable to reschedule before the expiration date listed on her paperwork and believed that was the end of her Medicaid coverage. Fearful that a continued lack of access to contraception would result in another unintended pregnancy, she made an appointment in Juárez to get an IUD.

Although Jazmine likely continued to have coverage according to Texas Medicaid records, the bureaucratic measures that resulted in her believing she had lost coverage meant she navigated health services as if she were uninsured. Like Jazmine, Alma also believed her Medicaid had expired when she began experiencing severe headaches and other concerning symptoms of high blood pressure. Believing she did not have coverage, she delayed seeking care. When she applied for the public hospital's discount program, she discovered she did in fact still have Medicaid coverage and was able to seek the care she needed. Such delays, however, can pose significant health threats. Headaches are typically not a symptom of high blood pressure until it has reached a level classified as a hypertensive crisis, putting a person at immediate risk of stroke or heart attack. To put it bluntly, Alma's delay in seeking care put her life in danger.

Elsewhere, I use the term *bureaucratic violence* to describe the ways that health care bureaucracy contributes to harm (Heckert 2020). Bureaucratic violence builds on the concept of legal violence. Legal violence emphasizes that the law can have far-reaching harmful effects for members of specific groups (Menjívar and Abrego 2012). Bureaucratic violence brings attention to the ways that it is not always the law itself that causes harm but rather the enactment of law via bureaucracy. Some laws, at face value, are not exclusionary. However, the enactment of policies can generate exclusion. During the pandemic, technically, Texas was not dropping anyone from Medicaid. Yet, bureaucratic mechanisms led to what Heide Castañeda (2019) describes as bureaucratic disentitlement, or de facto exclusion as administrative procedures prevented people from accessing the care to which they were entitled. The result was that people delayed or avoided seeking care that public programs should have covered.

A person's positionality may contribute to different experiences of bureaucratic violence. For those with Medicaid, there was a perception of loss of coverage. Those with CHIP Perinatal at times had profound fears over how the bureaucratic monitoring involved in using health programs could complicate immigration applications. This at times led to an avoidance of using publicly funded programs, including CHIP Perinatal. Legal ambiguities allow for multiple interpretations of the law (Das 2004). As such, changing bureaucratic procedures does not necessarily require a change in law. This facilitates the state's ability to subvert legislative processes and exert power (and harm) via bureaucracy. Bureaucratic changes to immigration laws, especially during the Donald Trump administration, contributed to the ways people made decisions about using CHIP Perinatal and other publicly funded programs. In particular, from 2018 to 2019, proposed changes to the likely public charge rule led some people to avoid using this program or express anxiety over using it. The likely public charge rule instructs immigration officials to deny a residency or naturalization application on the grounds that a person would be likely to use publicly funded programs. Between 1996 and 2018, USCIS guidelines stated that noncash benefits, including nutrition and health care programs, should not be used to deny an immigration application. In 2018, the Trump administration proposed changes to the rule that would result in use of noncash benefit programs as grounds for denying an application. While the final policy changes did make exceptions for using CHIP Perinatal and WIC, for over a year it was unclear what exactly the new public charge rule would entail. My 2018–19 research began after the announcement of proposed changes but before the release of the final guidelines. This marked a period of heightened uncertainty over the long-term implications of using CHIP Perinatal. A CNM who worked in both a hospital setting and community clinics explained her observations of how the fear of policy changes was shaping utilization of CHIP Perinatal. She said:

> It became very dramatically noticeable that after the election [of Trump] that people who are residing in the United States full time have become fearful to apply for CHIP. Many of those people are telling me that legal aid or lawyers are specifically telling them not to apply because it could affect future applications for residency or citizenship. Patients who I've seen previously at [the prenatal clinic associated with the public hospital], because they had CHIP, are now in community clinics paying by visit or getting some sort of discount there. It's not like it used to be when we would recommend you apply for CHIP and then people would go and apply for CHIP.

In 2018, I met Veronica at a community clinic when she was five months pregnant. Years prior, she had moved to El Paso to escape economic insecurity in Juárez. She expressed concern that applying for CHIP Perinatal could prevent her from being able to adjust her immigration status. She had two US-born teenagers. The oldest would be twenty-one years old soon, upon which she could sponsor her mother's immigration petition. At the time of our interview, Veronica was debating whether to apply for CHIP Perinatal. For the time being, she was paying ten dollars per visit at the community clinic, where she received care from a CNM. Given that Veronica had just turned forty, she believed she should be getting additional exams her midwife recommended, but the exams were a financial burden. She explained, "I went to inform myself about doing the sonogram, and they [at the doctor's office] told me no [about paying later]. I would have to pay upfront, and it was very expensive. But I have to do it." At the time, she was scrambling for money to pay for prenatal care rather than apply for CHIP Perinatal, not wanting to risk anything that could impact her ability to adjust her immigration status in the future. Reports of the proposed changes to the likely public charge rule may have exacerbated Veronica's concerns over using publicly funded care. However, it is also important to consider that immigrant communities already had preexisting fears over using publicly funded health programs, given that applicants must reveal their immigration status (Horton, Duncan, and Yarris 2018).

Sara, who migrated to the United States from Juárez using a tourist visa three years prior to our interview in 2018, shared experiences that suggested Veronica had legitimate fears. Sara moved to the United States primarily because her US-citizen husband convinced her to relocate after he was no longer able to cross the border after receiving probation following a drug-related offense. After the move, her husband became abusive and used her immigration status to control her. He also never sponsored her application for permanent residency, which he had promised to do. With the support of a local organization, she left him after giving birth to their child and applied for an adjustment of status through provisions under the Violence Against Women Act (VAWA). VAWA allows survivors of intimate partner violence to self-petition for legal residency if they were married to a US citizen or permanent resident. Shortly after submitting her application, the Trump administration announced plans to expand the likely public charge definition. Since Sara had used CHIP Perinatal during her pregnancy, her lawyer advised her that she might have problems with her adjustment of status. After receiving her temporary work permit, which USCIS typically grants while an application for permanent residency is under review, Sara had wanted to go to Juárez to visit family. She expressed confusion over her lawyer's advice to avoid going anywhere that would require her to pass through Border Patrol checkpoints, saying, "I don't know, the lawyer told us that we cannot go to Juárez because, because when they check the visas that it will appear that I was on CHIP and then they would not let me enter." The lawyer's advice to not leave El Paso compounded Sara's sense of entrapment (Núñez-Mchiri and Heyman 2007). Apart from not being able to travel beyond Border Patrol checkpoints, Sara also took a different route home every day, fearful her ex might be following her.

The legal definition of a likely public charge is ambiguous, and the execution of the law via bureaucratic procedures can enable the law to cause harm. The threat of expanding the definition of likely public charge as a grounds for denying immigration petitions illustrates how health care bureaucracy remains a potential extension of immigration enforcement. Bureaucratic measures that led Medicaid recipients to believe they no longer had access to coverage reflect another means through which bureaucracy can generate exclusion and result in adverse health outcomes. While a person's immigration status and type of health care coverage created different types of bureaucratic exclusion, ultimately, both publicly funded prenatal programs have the potential to generate harm via bureaucracy.

Historical Legacies of Being Uninsured

Salma's challenges in navigating postpartum care are a part of her longer history of exclusion from health care services. As a US-citizen child growing up in conditions of dire poverty in South Texas, she likely qualified for coverage under CHIP. However, her mother and older sister lacked legal status, which Salma said gave her mother a "fear of not being able to attain citizenship because you went and put your kids on government anything." She went on to explain:

> We needed food stamps. We could have gotten it. We qualified. Like neither of them [her mother and stepfather] was gainfully employed. I think they got maybe a thousand dollars between the two of them a month, and we were a family of, let's see, there's four kids and two of them. Six. They could have easily gotten assistance and gotten us better care. My mom was an immigrant, and afraid it was gonna affect her status when she wanted to become a citizen. That was a fear. Just her being deported. And the thing is, these things are offered. Like free asthma clinics.

Asthma was but one of the many childhood health ailments Salma suffered, as she also described being anemic throughout her childhood and early adulthood due to malnutrition, various forms of child abuse and neglect, severe allergies, and, later, diabetes. Of her allergies, she described learning that she was allergic to mice and cockroach feces, or in other words, was "allergic to being poor."

Despite these health ailments, she rarely saw doctors. Her mother often waited until a condition escalated before seeking care for her children. Salma provided an example: "When I was twelve, I got so bad that one of my cousins was like, 'If you don't take her to the emergency room, we're going to have to call the police on you.' And that's like the only way we ever really got seen was if somebody was like criticizing my mom, and it was always like emergency room services, never like regular care." Even as an adult, Salma described a tendency to avoid seeking health services. She explained, "From growing up that way, I have always avoided it [health care]," suggesting that she had developed a mindset of being uninsured by default. A lifetime of exclusion from health services had led her to act as if she were uninsured, even during periods of her life when she gained coverage. Her assumption that she would once again lack insurance following her pregnancy may have contributed to her interpreting her Medicaid renewal form as an expiration notice.

Many people with coverage under Medicaid for Pregnant Women have experienced different degrees of exclusion from health services—and various forms of social marginalization that undergird this health exclusion—throughout their life course. Temporary inclusion in care during pregnancy cannot remedy historical injustices. The lack of remediation contributes to epidemiological patterns that show more adverse birth and postpartum outcomes among pregnancies covered by Medicaid (Dang et al. 2011).

Of course, not all pregnancies covered by Medicaid involve people who have faced a lifetime of blocked access to healthcare. One group that often uses this program is young adults who have recently lost insurance after aging out of CHIP or losing coverage under a parent's plan. Many individuals who had private insurance or Tricare, which is an insurance program through the military, in the past speculated that recent experiences of disregard or outright mistreatment by providers stemmed from the fact that they had Medicaid. For example, we interviewed Lorena during her fourth pregnancy, which was the first pregnancy she carried to term. She had previously experienced two miscarriages and a second trimester intrauterine fetal demise during her third pregnancy. Terrified that she would never be able to carry a pregnancy to term, she requested further tests to figure out what was causing the miscarriages. She described having to go through several doctors before finding someone who was willing to run additional tests. When asked why she thought she had these challenges finding care, she said, "Well, I think I expected it since I was on Medicaid, and it [her health care] was just covered by the government health benefits. Then when I started working at the Post Office, I got their insurance, and they were kind of more motivated to do tests on me. I did see a difference."

Those covered by CHIP Perinatal also had multiple degrees of access to health services outside of pregnancy. Length of time living in the United States, ability to cross the US-Mexico border for services in Mexico, and ability to navigate local safety-net programs and community clinics contributed to patterns in lifetime access to care within this group.

Adelaide had protections and a work permit under DACA but had otherwise been undocumented since her family relocated to El Paso when she was seven years old in order to flee violence in Juárez. Like Salma, she spent her childhood with extremely limited access to health care, describing never going to the doctor, unless it was an emergency or required for school. Similar to Salma, in developing a mentality of being uninsured, she often ignored health issues until an illness or pain became severe. Luckily, being in her early twenties, she felt like she was fairly healthy and had few health concerns. However, she expressed a desire for different forms of care, which included a prepregnancy consultation given a past miscarriage and a way to access contraception, expressing concern that she would become pregnant again too quickly following the birth. Without documentation, she could not cross to Mexico for these services. Hypothetically, she could access birth control through a community clinic, although she was unaware this service was available at the clinics she had visited in the past.

Like Adelaide, Sandra had DACA and was covered under CHIP Perinatal. Spending most of her life without health insurance, Sandra had learned to navigate local programs that could offer some access to health services. In Sandra's case, she faced more immediate health risks than Adelaide if she did not access care. She had already given birth twice, and following her second pregnancy, she developed type 2 diabetes. While she was able to manage the diabetes without medication in the earlier stages, her condition required monitoring and she eventually needed medication. After applying for the discount program through the local public hospital, she was able to visit a specialist for twenty-four dollars and obtain her medications for eight dollars—prices that were affordable to her. The differences in Adelaide's and Sandra's experiences demonstrate how a person's ability to navigate local safety-net programs also factors into stratified access.

Many people with CHIP Perinatal did have somewhat stable access to health services outside of pregnancy through their ability to use services across the border. Liliana was a thirty-one-year-old permanent resident who initially came to El Paso with a student visa that allowed her to easily cross back and forth from Juárez. Shortly after graduating, she applied for residency via marriage to a US citizen. As a child, given that her parents had stable middle class employment, she consistently had access to the private health sector in Mexico. As a student, she simply crossed to Juárez when she needed health services. After graduating, she at times had private insurance, but when she lost this coverage, she maintained her pattern of using more affordable services in Mexico. Liliana's health seeking strategies are common on the border, although much less feasible for those with CHIP Perinatal residing outside of the border region. Further, it is also a strategy that requires some degree of economic resources to utilize private doctors and a legal immigration status in order to freely cross.

Although those with CHIP Perinatal had more limited coverage to the US health system than those with Medicaid, people often described care under CHIP Perinatal in more favorable terms. Much of this stemmed from feeling like the quality of care in the US was better than the quality of care in Mexico. This was especially true of women who had given birth within the Mexican public sector, where experiences of obstetric violence are widespread (Castro and Erviti 2014). Flor had previous birth experiences in both Mexico and the United States and explained her preference for giving birth in the United States: "[In the United States,] they treat you better. In other words, you have more care with the pregnancy, and someone is with the mother. They give you more attention during the birth process and don't leave you alone. In Mexico, it's not like that." Brisa, whose birth experience I discussed in the introduction, described feeling like she had a "harmonious birth," despite numerous complications. She attributed this to feeling like her midwife was attentive and gentle, in comparison to how providers in rural Mexico had treated her. However, not all women with CHIP Perinatal felt like they received optimal care and, like those with Medicaid, often attributed this to the type of coverage that they had. For example, while seeking care for a miscarriage, Adelaide felt like providers at a private hospital treated her poorly. Emergency room staff left her alone in a room and denied her request for pain medication, despite the severe levels of pain she reported.

There were multiple historical trajectories of access to care among women covered by CHIP Perinatal and Medicaid. While these programs are a reflection of stratified access during pregnancy, stratified access throughout the life course was more complex than simply the type of prenatal and birth coverage a person had. Immigration histories, structural vulnerabilities, and ability to cross the border to seek services in Mexico are among the factors that contribute to various degrees of inclusion and exclusion from care among those included under both programs.

Publicly Funded Care as Limiting Bodily Autonomy

Liliana had her first child in May 2020. Two months prior to the birth, the City of El Paso issued stay-at-home orders in response to the growing threat from COVID-19. The threat from COVID-19 spurred Liliana to quit her job out of fear of contracting the virus while pregnant. This was not a difficult decision, given that she was already planning to take a break from work following the birth and she had coverage for her prenatal care and birth through her husband's health insurance. However, this coverage only lasted through her first month postpartum, as her husband lost his job in the middle of widespread layoffs due to the pandemic. Only having recently gained permanent residency status in 2019, Liliana had no way to access Healthy Texas Women to cover birth control. She thought that breastfeeding would at least temporarily protect her from getting pregnant, but six months postpartum, she became pregnant again.

While Liliana did eventually want another child, the timing was not ideal for her. Her family had experienced a set of financial setbacks. Just after securing a new job, her husband fell ill with COVID-19. Given he would be paid commission, the missed work meant it would be at least several weeks before they would see a paycheck. As bills piled up, the coupled borrowed money from family to cover rent and groceries. When Liliana discovered she was pregnant again, her husband decided to take a job working in the oil fields a four-hour-drive away. This decision came with a sacrifice to family unity and left Liliana alone and with the baby for long stretches during her second pregnancy, but they saw it as their only option to make enough money to pay back family members and support a growing family.

Given that Liliana's husband was still unemployed when she initially sought prenatal care, she qualified for CHIP Perinatal. While she felt this program was sufficient for covering her prenatal care and birth, it provided no postpartum coverage for birth control. Following the birth of her second baby, Liliana was adamant about starting birth control right away. However, her lack of coverage constrained her decision about what type of birth control to use. She had initially wanted to get the implant but explained: "I found out that [CHIP Perinatal] wouldn't cover any type of contraceptive. The shot was the cheapest and the safest. The shot was eighty-five [dollars] I think, and it's every three months and I thought I can afford that. Because the implant is over $3,000." Given that Liliana had expressed a preference for the implant, at her postpartum visit, her provider gave her information on a community clinic that offered birth control on a sliding scale. However, Liliana never followed up, believing that since her husband had gained stable employment, she would not qualify for help. She said, "I scheduled an appointment for an interview with them, but I ended up canceling it because my husband was getting paid enough. I had to take pay stubs and show them. They were going to be like, 'He is doing good. Why can't you afford it?' Well, I can't afford it since I have other debts," referring to the money they had borrowed while unemployed.

Liliana's struggle to access birth control shows how the policies that result in limited access to health services have implications for a person's ability to control the timing of their pregnancies. As Liliana's experiences show, this struggle was particularly acute for those with CHIP Perinatal, as those with Medicaid could typically access Healthy Texas Women. However, those who could have qualified for Healthy Texas Women often reported they were not aware of this program until after becoming pregnant. Consequently, roughly half of participants reported that their most recent pregnancy was unplanned. Anahí, who had Medicaid, described her experience with birth control access: "Like I never have been on birth control or any things like that. No, I have never, like I never even heard of anything. I didn't know there was places like that teen center, or stuff like that, you know? Until I became pregnant. Then everyone was like, 'There is one here, and there is one here,' and I am like, 'Really?' I didn't know there were so many until I became pregnant. I really had like no idea actually."

When women had an unplanned pregnancy, it often limited their sense of autonomy in various ways. Susana, who was undocumented and had CHIP Perinatal, reported being unsure of how to access contraception without health insurance. Her unplanned fourth pregnancy took a significant toll on her mental health since she had to stop working and felt extremely isolated staying home all day after thinking she was done having children. Similarly, Rebecca had not planned her most recent pregnancy and said she would be "suicidal" if she were to get pregnant again. Since she was a US citizen, she could access Healthy Texas Women after her Medicaid expired. Through that program, she planned to get a copper IUD, since, in the past, her body had not reacted well to hormonal birth control.

Providers commented on how limitations on access to birth control shaped the types of contraception individuals sought out as well as the forms of birth control they encouraged among their patients. A CNM reported that some patients with CHIP Perinatal who knew that they were going to have a C-section would request having their tubes tied as an add-on procedure. Knowing these individuals may struggle to access birth control, providers were quick to oblige. Margot, an undocumented woman with CHIP Perinatal, made this request. Since her first child was an emergency C-section, she was having a planned C-section for her second child and knew she did not want more children.

Aside from supporting decisions about sterilization, providers may also be quick to encourage long-acting reversible contraception (LARC), such as an IUD, among low-income people of color (Dehlendorf et al. 2010). While this pattern may arise from concerns that this group has barriers to securing other forms of birth control, individual decisions to use LARC or undergo sterilization may be a consequence of constraints rather than preference, thus showing the ways lack of coverage limits the degree of autonomy people have over their bodies (López 2008; Moniz et al. 2017). As Iris López (2008) shows, reproductive decisions are never purely about individual desires, as social circumstances, interpersonal relationships, and gender inequalities always have a bearing on the viability of different options. When women choose sterilization or LARC, they may be making a choice under oppressive circumstances, which puts into question the degree of choice marginalized populations are able to exercise.

While some women felt LARC was ideal, others reported hesitations to use such methods because of challenges in removing devices when they did want to get pregnant. Magdalena, a US citizen whose Medicaid was about to expire following the birth of her child in 2018, described her preferred form of birth control: "I think the IUD, but if it wasn't so long term. It is like three years or something, so I wish they had like an annual thing. And that the removal wouldn't have an extra cost to take it out. Does that make sense? You can take it off anytime, but I think they do charge you for it." Magdalena's considerations for how she could get an IUD removed without health insurance emphasizes how use of LARC may address short-term concerns about limited access to birth control but has a long-term consequence of continuing to prevent pregnancy when people may actively want to get pregnant. While Magdalena may have had power in choosing an IUD, it was a choice made in a context of limited options for an acceptable form of birth control.

People's perspectives on the forms of birth control most readily available to them echo what Lina-Maria Murillo (2021) describes as a historical legacy of the paradox of coercion and choice in the region. As in other parts of the United States, the first birth control clinics in El Paso garnered support through eugenics discourses that generated fears among whites that Black and Brown people would continue to reproduce and outnumber whites. In the borderlands, Anglos viewed people of Mexican origin as a racial threat, but a blue- and pink-collar Mexican workforce was also an economic necessity. As a consequence, the regional goal was to control reproduction, rather than stop it. As such, Texas was reluctant to adopt policies that led to forced sterilizations, in contrast to other states where this practice was widespread (see Vélez-Ibáñez 1980). Instead, state and local health programs engaged in efforts to expand the use of experimental birth control among Mexican-origin women. Despite the use of potentially coercive tactics and making Brown bodies the subjects of experimentation, Murillo (2021) also shows that Mexican-origin women heavily utilized early birth control clinics in El Paso to gain control over their reproductive lives.

Availability of different services in the United States and Mexico also enables some people to have additional choices if they are able to cross the border. People traveling from the US side of the border have long used providers in Mexico to terminate pregnancies, especially during points in history when abortion has been illegal in the United States. Although Mexico did not decriminalize abortion until 2021, historically, there has been weak enforcement of abortion laws. As a result, prior to *Roe v. Wade*, people residing in the United States and desiring an abortion utilized social networks to find providers in Mexico willing to perform the procedure (Murillo 2016).

The topic of abortion did not come up often in interviews. This may be in large part because of how we structured the research. In recruiting pregnant people, inclusion criteria included people who were past the first trimester to limit attrition due to miscarriage or abortion. We did interview some individuals who mentioned considering abortion but had ultimately decided to continue with the pregnancy. It seems that those who found themselves in a situation of a forced pregnancy may have been more likely to self-select out of participating in an interview. For example, one person who participated in the survey phase of our research reported a high degree of emotional distress and, in open-ended responses to questions on the emotional distress scale, stated "not wanting to be pregnant" as the cause of these emotions. However, this person declined to participate in a follow-up interview, preventing us from understanding what factors led her to continue the pregnancy.

Despite the lack of interview discussion on abortion, it is important to consider the role of shifting abortion policies during the timeframe of this research. On September 1, 2021, Texas Senate Bill 8 (SB-8) went into effect, banning abortions once a sonogram could detect fetal cardiac activity, which typically occurs at six weeks' gestation—which is often before a person even knows they are pregnant. This legislation does not use the state to enforce the law, instead allowing any private citizen to sue an individual for "aiding and abetting" an abortion, working around the protections granted under *Roe v. Wade* that still existed at the time. Following the Supreme Court overturn of *Roe v. Wade*, Texas's trigger law went into effect, which makes providing an abortion a felony that can result in life in prison.

Of course, abortions are continuing to occur for anyone who is able to access the resources to travel out of state or use telehealth services to seek a medicated abortion. In the border region, there is also the possibility of self-managing an abortion by obtaining drugs easily available without a prescription in Mexico. Poor and disenfranchised communities with less access to these resources will continue to bear the burden of lack of access to safe abortions. Providing some degree of relief for those wishing to terminate a pregnancy in El Paso is the geographic proximity to New Mexico and Mexico. While El Paso has a geographically large urban sprawl, the western edge of the city bleeds into New Mexico, a state that has maintained access to abortion care without gestational limits.

Lina was one of the few participants who spoke in-depth about considering an abortion and would have had to travel to New Mexico for the procedure. At her twenty-week sonogram, her doctor discovered the baby had hydrocephaly, a condition characterized by fluid buildup in the brain. It is often the consequence of an underlying condition, such as spina bifida or other spinal cord abnormalities. Because of these associated conditions, hydrocephaly is often related to other developmental challenges and disabilities. However, the full diagnosis is uncertain at twenty weeks' gestation. While Lina never thought she would have considered an abortion, she was unsure if she was ready to raise a child whose diagnosis was still unclear. Ultimately, she decided to continue with the pregnancy. Before doing so, she scheduled an appointment in Albuquerque, New Mexico, an over five-hundred-mile round-trip drive from El Paso and the closest location of a clinic that could perform an abortion well into the second trimester. Lina was in a situation where she could have made this trip if she decided to terminate the pregnancy. She was a US-born citizen and did not have to fear crossing an internal Border Patrol checkpoint that would prevent an undocumented person from making this trip. While Medicaid would not have covered any of her costs, financially, she felt stable enough to afford the costs associated with travel.

Apart from traveling to another US state, one can also walk to Juárez, Mexico, from downtown El Paso. While the Mexican Supreme Court decriminalized abortion less than a week after SB-8 went into effect, it created a grey zone by allowing states to decide whether abortions are fully legal. The state of Chihuahua, where Juárez is located, has not legalized abortion. However, misoprostol is readily available at Mexican pharmacies without a prescription. Even when abortion was more accessible in Texas, use of misoprostol from a Mexican pharmacy was often easier to access and more private (Reed-Sandoval 2022). For a pregnant person who has access to correct information about the dosage and timing necessary for a self-managed abortion with medication, misoprostol effectively terminates a first-trimester pregnancy about 80 percent of the time (Speer 2019). When used alongside mifepristone, the effectiveness increases to about 95 percent (Donovan 2018). However, mifepristone is not easily available in Mexico, meaning that people procuring abortion medication in Mexico have a less than ideal regime by relying on misoprostol alone. Use of misoprostol typically causes cramping and bleeding, even if the pregnancy has not been fully terminated. With access to only part of the full abortion medication combination and with potentially limited follow-up care, an unsuccessful abortion attempt may lead to the continuation of an unwanted pregnancy or subsequent abortion attempts occurring at a later stage in the pregnancy.

Medicaid and CHIP Perinatal both generated constraints for exercising reproductive autonomy, as these programs limit access to ideal forms of birth control, which has implications for maintaining control over the timing of pregnancies. This is occurring against a backdrop of state legislation that is increasingly limiting access to abortion, which disproportionately burdens economically disadvantaged populations that utilize publicly funded prenatal care. The geographic location of El Paso mediates access for some people but this access is contingent upon immigration status and ability to travel across borders and internal border checkpoints.

Health Policy as Reproductive Violence

The narratives of people utilizing CHIP Perinatal and Medicaid demonstrate how health care policies and legislation can function as reproductive violence. Women covered under both programs suffered significant harms beyond the realm of clinical encounters, as bureaucratic violence prevented them from even engaging with health services. For those with CHIP Perinatal, there was the added effect of legal exclusion from health services. In such cases, health policy contributed to medical negligence, or the failure to provide appropriate care. The US health care system systematically generates medical negligence through the exclusion of those without coverage, ultimately leading to harm. While this exclusion is often blatant, other times it is more invisible, such as when bureaucratic mechanisms lead to exclusion. Although the system itself is negligent, the legal avenues for making claims of medical negligence are designed to hold individual practitioners, rather than the entire system, accountable. As a consequence, legal remedies only exist when a person has access to care to begin with. The lack of recourse that people have when harmed perpetuates the invisibility of widespread negligence and the persistence of harm. By describing this negligent system as a primary source of reproductive violence, my goal is to emphasize the ways that the health care system itself, and policies that lead to widespread exclusion from care, manifest as maternal harm.

Many people described experiences of exclusion throughout their life course. This is in large part a function of health care policies that value a woman's womb over the entirety of her bodily health. As people struggled to access the care they needed outside of the temporary period of pregnancy, many of their health needs went unaddressed, setting them up for riskier pregnancies that involve more interventions and adverse outcomes. People with CHIP Perinatal may not even have access to the care they need while pregnant, given that this program does not provide comprehensive coverage. Further, temporary inclusion in care cannot remedy a lifetime of health care exclusion and other forms of injustice that make a person vulnerable to ill health. Additionally, limited access to contraception significantly constrained individuals' abilities to control the circumstances and timing of their pregnancies.

Texas may be on the verge of extending care postpartum for those with Medicaid, yet the way the state bureaucratically managed continuous Medicaid coverage during the public health emergency illustrates some of the substantial barriers that prevent people from fully utilizing the care they may need and to which they are entitled. In the midst of discussion of postpartum Medicaid extension, people with CHIP Perinatal remain nearly completely excluded from postpartum care in the United States that is needed to address what may escalate into a life-threatening condition. Further, as reference to maternal mortality and severe morbidity dominates policy discussions, it is also important to consider the ways that less quantifiable forms of harm, such as Anessa's loss of her ability to breastfeed due to untreated mastitis, are likely not registered in databases of adverse birth outcomes.

2

Immigration Policy and Embodied Vulnerabilities

When Marla became pregnant with her first child in 2008, she was in her third year of taking classes part-time at a community college while working to support herself. The unplanned pregnancy thwarted her plans to transfer to a four-year university to complete a bachelor's degree. Despite having to put this goal on hold, she initially felt like things would work out. Her boyfriend Efraín promised to support her and the baby so that she could quickly return to school. Although Efraín's undocumented status limited his job prospects, he had steady income working construction jobs as a welder. The couple also decided to marry, and Marla hoped her status as a US-born citizen would enable her to sponsor Efraín's application for permanent residency. However, when they sought legal counsel, their lawyer advised them to abandon the application. Efraín had a past deportation on his record. In the process of applying for residency, immigration policies at the time would require him to exit the United States. Upon attempted return, his past deportation would trigger a ban on reentry.

Following this disappointment, Marla went into labor eight weeks early. Her son, born prematurely, also had a low birth weight and required weeks in the NICU (neonatal intensive care unit). During labor, Marla's blood pressure began to spike to dangerous levels and her OB-GYN (doctor of obstetrics and gynecology) informed her she had preeclampsia. When the baby was only six months old, Marla said, "Then it all happened, like, he [Efraín] got deported. He was going to work one day, and he had his boss pick him up at an RV. I guess since it was like the third day that they were meeting there, someone called the Border Patrol." Following the deportation, Efraín faced a ten-year ban from entering the United States.

After Efraín's deportation, Marla spent time living in Juárez when she could, for the sake of family unity. However, the couple primarily maintained a cross-border relationship. Marla's citizenship status enabled her to cross regularly to Juárez to see her husband. At the time of our interview in early 2019, Efraín's ban on reentry had ended and they were awaiting a response on their petition for his US residency. Marla had also recently given birth to their second child. The couple had wanted to be living together before having another child, but Marla experienced a birth control failure and unexpectedly got pregnant. She found her second pregnancy more stressful than the first, and she worried the stress would be bad for the baby. She said:

> My whole pregnancy was stressful. I had to go to Mexico, and coming back, the lines are always long. It's like the heat, and then I was so big. I had to keep working. I couldn't stop working 'cause I already had my son. It was a very stressful experience. I had high blood pressure. They were always on the lookout for that during my pregnancy. I guess it was all the stress that I went through, 'cause like I said, I had to keep working, and then I had to go over there. Like, even though it was my day off, I still had to like go over there. I couldn't stay here and just rest. Like I had to go over there cause my son, he's always been attached to his dad, so he always wanted to go, so I couldn't say no. But yeah, I had high blood pressure. During the labor, the blood pressure spiked like very high, and I guess that's the reason why my baby was born with respiratory distress, cause the higher my blood pressure would go, the less oxygen she could receive.

Making her birth experience even more difficult was the fact that her husband, still banned from the United States, could not be at the hospital with her for the birth or the three days that their second child was in the NICU. The experience of being separated from a partner or other loved ones for the birth became much more prevalent among transnational families during the long-term closure of the border during the pandemic. Yet, Marla's account demonstrates that border and immigration policies have always generated hardships by dividing families.

Marla's account reflects two broader themes among people who had immigrated to the United States or had loved ones who were immigrants: first, immigration-related concerns played a central role in producing emotional distress, even among women with a secure immigration status and, second, resulting emotions were frequently cited as a cause of maternal health risks and birth complications. In exploring the relationship among immigration-related concerns, emotional distress, and maternal and infant health outcomes, I return to embodiment theory and how it relates to local biologies.

The Embodiment of Immigration Policy

Embodiment refers to the ways social processes become incorporated into bodily experience (Csordas 1993; Gravlee 2009; Krieger 2016; Willen 2007). Analyzing experiences of emotional distress can deepen understandings of embodiment as a complex, multilevel process (Downey 2014; Hinton 1999; Willen 2012). Emotional distress includes negative emotional reactions, or the psychological dimensions of stress, resulting from stressors in the social environment. Stress includes both subjective emotional experiences and bodily responses to perceived or actual threats (Lazarus 1999). As epidemiological research shows, social stressors and the subsequent stress response are a primary pathway through which social injustice translates into health disparities, as the stress response stimulates bodily reactions that can have negative health implications, especially if stress is chronic (Campbell and Ehlert 2012). The emotions resulting from stressful circumstances cue the physiological stress response, which helps explain how emotions generate health vulnerabilities. However, emotional experiences are not always easy to predict for epidemiological analysis. As women's narratives show, emotional responses to immigration-related concerns are subjective and relational. Women may experience immigration policies and the social disadvantages they produce in multiple ways that contribute to emotional distress. The narratives in this chapter highlight the role of time, place, and social relationships in shaping emotional experiences in response to immigration-related issues. In the US-Mexico border region, patterns of increased border militarization combined with a heavily Latino population, where mixed-immigration-status households are common, may generate a burden of stress that manifests in *local biologies*. Conceptually, the idea of local biologies links biological processes to the particularities of a specific context, attending to how the political climate, structural constraints, cultural norms, and environmental factors shape vulnerability to and experiences of conditions

(Lock 1993). The concept of local biologies elucidates how the border context may be contributing to epidemiological patterns and the experience of certain conditions. Epidemiological patterns related to maternal and infant health along the Texas-Mexico border are distinct from those at the state and national levels. Marla's experiences with preterm birth and preeclampsia reflect a localized pattern characterized by higher prevalence rates of these conditions (Patel et al. 2017).

Women's narratives point to a need to carefully analyze the ways individual histories and different types of immigration-related apprehensions can shape embodied health vulnerabilities in a highly militarized border context. I do so using women's perceptions of what contributed to their health risks during pregnancy, as women's explanatory models often link their social worlds to ill health (Finkler 1994; Gálvez 2011; Tapias 2015). To explore the ways women perceive emotional distress resulting from immigration-related concerns as affecting their health, I analyze women's experiences in relation to the *embodiment of immigration-related precarity*, *corporeal kinship effects of immigration*, and *embodied histories of immigration-related vulnerability*. The embodiment of immigration-related precarity refers to how one's own immigration status generates exclusion. Corporeal kinship effects of immigration arise because, even if a woman has a secure immigration status, immigration concerns over loved ones may generate stress. The discussion of embodied histories of immigration-related vulnerability draws attention to how one's immigration status is subject to change. Even if a woman feels secure, a history of being undocumented may have generated past experiences of emotional distress with long-lasting physiological consequences.

Explanatory Models of Emotional Distress and Embodied Vulnerability

Anahí, a second-generation immigrant, had not planned her pregnancy. However, when she discovered she was pregnant in early 2018, Anahí and her boyfriend were happy about having a baby. Anahí's boyfriend planned to move in with her and her parents around the time of the birth. Just before the move, he went to Juárez to help his father with a job, had his US permanent residency card stolen, and was unable to return to El Paso until United States Citizenship and Immigration Services (USCIS) accepted his application for a replacement card. This took months, given that he had to come up with the $540 fee to submit the application. In the meantime, Anahí was thirty-eight-weeks pregnant when her provider informed her that they would need to induce labor. Although Anahí stated that her OB-GYN never gave her a clear explanation of why he wanted to induce labor, she felt like she did not have a choice. Following induction, her labor progressed slowly. When her cervix had not fully dilated after twenty-four hours, her OB-GYN informed her they would be moving to a C-section.[1] Her boyfriend missed the birth, making it back to El Paso when the baby was a week old.

Anahí reported feeling nervous and stressed as she anxiously waited for her boyfriend's return. In fact, she had felt stressed throughout her entire pregnancy. This was in part because she had been arguing with her boyfriend frequently but also, more importantly to her, because she dreaded going to her job at a grocery store everyday where her supervisor constantly harassed her. Anahí, like many women we interviewed, did her best to control her emotions, worried that negative emotions could harm the baby. She explained:

> My mom kept telling me, "Don't let it affect you too much because [the baby] feels everything, and when she comes out, she will be a stressful baby." Because I had a cousin who was pregnant and had a really horrible pregnancy, because I think her significant other died. So yeah, her baby came out, and there is nothing really wrong with her, but she is just a little off. . . . Everybody kept saying it was because of the stress she had. So I was thinking, "My daughter is going to come out, and something is going to be wrong with her."

Arthur Kleinman and colleagues (1978) describe an explanatory model as encompassing the social meaning a person attaches to a condition, including causes of ill health. As Anahí explained the connections between her emotions and her baby's health, she was offering her explanatory model of how stress may cause adverse birth outcomes. Although Anahí had a failed induction that resulted in a C-section, she reported a healthy birth. However, throughout her pregnancy, she feared her emotions could cause something to go wrong. This explanatory model that views emotional distress during pregnancy as a potential cause of harm has been documented among Mexican immigrants (see Gálvez 2011), and we found similar explanations among US-born citizens of Mexican descent, including Anahí.

The medical literature substantiates Anahí's explanatory model that stress can generate negative birth outcomes (Dunkel Schetter and Glynn 2011). While the relationship between maternal stress and birth outcomes is well documented, shifting attention to women's subjective experiences more clearly shows how the social context translates into health vulnerability. Past research suggests that a precarious immigration status does not necessarily correlate with poorer health outcomes (Hummer et al. 2007). The emotions women experience in response to policies, and their perceptions of how these emotions produce health vulnerabilities, can show why polices have varied and sometimes unpredictable outcomes, suggesting a need to interrogate what specifically about immigration status produces emotional distress.

In exploring how women perceived their emotions as contributing to health vulnerabilities, I analyze the experiences of a subgroup of women who we interviewed postpartum and who reported stress-sensitive health conditions, including preeclampsia, hypertensive conditions, diabetes, preterm birth, and low birth weight. Appendix III includes a table of women who we interviewed postpartum who reported at least one stress-sensitive health condition. The table also includes information about immigration-related concerns as well as other social stressors that women reported. The women included in the table are not the only ones who experienced emotional distress. Rather, emotional distress produced by immigration-related issues was common, although to varying degrees. Even among women with healthy births, such as Anahí, there was often worry that negative emotions could trigger negative outcomes. By foregrounding those who had adverse outcomes, my aim is to use women's explanatory models to illustrate how they connected their emotions to these health outcomes.

Embodiment of Immigration-Related Precarity

Leisy Abrego and Sarah Lakhani (2015) and Cecilia Menjívar (2006) operationalize a precarious immigration status as not having documentation or having a liminal status subject to expiration, making one deportable. Women's narratives, however, complicate notions of how immigration policy generates precarity. A precarious immigration status did not always translate into a lived sense of insecurity (although it often did), while having protection from deportation did not always prevent women from feeling insecure. For example, Lydia had overstayed the thirty consecutive days permitted in the United States using a border crossing card but described not feeling concerned about her immigration status. Although she had technically become undocumented, she had been in the Unites States for less than a year. If deported, she would return to Juárez, content her child was born in the United States and could return for greater opportunities. In comparison, Zahra had permanent residency and felt strong ties to the United States. She had married a US citizen with whom she had two children. Given she had been a permanent resident for less than five years, she expressed a sense of exclusion from resources such as food stamps and Medicaid, which have length of residency requirements for eligibility. These were resources she desperately needed during her most recent pregnancy in 2018, when her and her husband both lost their jobs, were evicted from their apartment, and lived out of their car until shortly before the birth. Thus, a sense of precarity was not neatly aligned with immigration status. One consistent pattern, however, was that when women felt vulnerability tied to being an immigrant, it often caused emotional distress.

Margot described how her undocumented immigration status generated insecurity. Margot had not wanted another child when she became pregnant with her second child. She already had a teenage son with DiGeorge syndrome and feared she would have another child with special needs. Although her daughter was healthy, her pregnancy was high risk with elevated blood pressure and gestational diabetes. She attributed both conditions to her stressful life as undocumented and caring for a child with special needs, saying, "At seven months, they diagnosed me with diabetes and told me the high blood pressure was because of so much stress. It wasn't stress from the pregnancy, but stress from a life with *nervios* [anxiety] and a stress that accumulates, from having a special needs child and, apart from that, not having papers. It is very stressful for you, because sometimes you don't sleep or eat.

Because you have a doctor's appointment you say, 'Immigration goes by there often. My God, what am I going to do?' and all of this, all of this is very stressful." Exacerbating Margot's anxiety was that the southern boundary of her neighborhood ends at the US-Mexico border wall. Border Patrol vehicles and helicopters are always present in the area. She described her reasons for living in her neighborhood, despite the constant reminders of immigration enforcement: "I live here because for one, the rent here is cheaper. Second, here all the buses take us to where I need to go, and I go everywhere on the bus. Third, about half of the people here are immigrants, so with this you feel more confident with the others. But on the other hand, it gives you *nervios* because you start to talk to someone, you turn around, and at your back you see *la migra* [immigration agents] coming, but you have to act like they don't make you nervous."

Margot highlighted how her undocumented status contributed to everyday experiences of emotional distress. She repeatedly referred to the relationship between *nervios* and stress. Although there are regional variations in defining *nervios*, it is commonly attributed to a social source of suffering that results in emotional and physical symptoms (Guarnaccia and Farias 1988). Beyond bodily ills, Margot's immigration status led her to monitor her own movements. She trained herself to act like the *migra* did not make her nervous so they would not become suspicious of her.

Some women experienced compounded sources of precarity, like Sofi, a survivor of intimate partner violence who was in the process of adjusting her immigration status and was pregnant with her third child in 2018. Sofi said, "For nineteen years, I have been fighting to get my papers." As a child, her mother and stepfather petitioned for her residency. According to Sofi, "Immigration kept messing up purposely because they kept sending documentation to the old address." In 2011, Sofi married a US citizen after becoming pregnant. She was hesitant to marry, given her partner's abusive past. However, they were living in a state without CHIP Perinatal, and her only option for accessing prenatal coverage was marriage so she could qualify for insurance under her husband's plan. Her decision to marry illustrates how health policies tied to immigration status shape *reproductive habitus* (Fleuriet and Sunil 2015; Smith-Oka 2012). Reproductive habitus includes "modes of living the reproductive body, bodily practices, and the creation of new subjects through interactions between people and structures" (Smith-Oka 2012, 2276). Sofi's perception that marriage was her only viable option for accessing prenatal care reflects the social inequities that excluded her from health services. The marriage may have resulted in access to insurance to mitigate the risks that come from not seeking prenatal care, but it put her at heightened risk of other forms of bodily harm at the hands of an abusive husband. Five days after Sofi married, she said her husband "beat me until my face was unrecognizable." After this incident, among many others, Sofi stayed with her husband in part because he was a US citizen, and she hoped he would sponsor her residency. After leaving him the first time, she felt pressured to return because of her immigration situation. She explained, "I packed, and I never looked back until I was in Georgia. We were there for four years, and the immigration lawyer was like, 'Well, since he is a US citizen, you should get back with him so that you can get your papers so that he can file for you and within three months you will get it.'" Sofi described how her immigration status contributed to her decision to stay in an unsafe situation, which is a broader pattern among battered immigrant women (Parson and Heckert 2014; Salcido and Adelman 2004). Sofi's now ex-husband never petitioned for her residency and, instead, the violence escalated. She described her decision to leave for good: "An incident broke out in 2016, and that's when he [attacked] me with a fire extinguisher. But when he swung, he missed me, but hit my son in the head. So, I called the cops, and we hopped on a bus and came to El Paso." After relocating, Sofi found support from a community organization that helped her apply for residency through provisions under the Violence Against Women Act (VAWA), which enables undocumented women in abusive relationships to self-petition for residency if married to a US citizen or permanent resident. In late 2018, Sofi was awaiting a decision on her adjustment of status application, had begun a new relationship, and was pregnant with her third child.

The intersection of immigration insecurities and an abusive relationship created multiple health vulnerabilities for Sofi and her children. Beyond the risks from physical violence, Sofi described how her emotions shaped her pregnancies and births:

You know, when a woman is pregnant for the first time, it is just like, "Whoa." It's just happiness. For me, it was just sadness. I was happy to be carrying a baby, but I was more concerned because how we feel during our pregnancy affects the kid. So, my son was five pounds when he was born, and days would go on, and he would not move. I was always concerned. Even with my daughter, the same thing. So, with this one, I am more, I am more happy about it because I am happy. With the other ones all I did was just cry. That's what I remember throughout my pregnancies. Just crying and just arguments.

Within Sofi's explanatory model, she believed her sadness contributed to her first two children having low birth weights. Having left the abusive relationship, she described happiness for her current pregnancy. With this happiness came what felt like a healthier pregnancy. This distinction emphasizes the significance Sofi placed on her emotions in shaping the health of her babies.

The extended closure of the US-Mexico border during the pandemic created an additional source of insecurity for some women with mixed-status transborder families. In nonpandemic times, some people residing in El Paso who are unable to freely cross the border because of their immigration status are able to see family members from the Mexican side if those family members have a border crossing card. During the border closure, US citizens and permanent residents could still freely cross the border by land, but those with a tourist visa or border crossing card could not.

Anessa profoundly felt the repercussions of being cut off from family members during the border closure. Prior to marrying a US citizen, Anessa and her family frequently crossed the border using border crossing cards. After her marriage, Anessa remained in El Paso while she awaited the approval of her permanent residency application. The extended closure of the border marked this timeframe, which resulted in Anessa going nearly her entire pregnancy without seeing her family members who could no longer come visit her in El Paso. Anessa reported intense depression during her pregnancy, which she attributed to feeling isolated and disconnected from her mother and sister.

As Margot and Sofi demonstrate, immigration status was often an important factor in producing a feeling of precarity. However, Lydia's sense of security despite her lack of legal status demonstrates the variability in emotions women experienced in relation to their immigration status. Lydia felt secure largely because she was a lifelong border resident and did not fear being deported only a short distance, while her US-citizen child would maintain the ability to freely cross the border. In this sense, the context of the border was protective. Other women expressed similar sentiments by explaining how even though they were immigrants, they felt welcome and included in El Paso because the city's population is bicultural and bilingual. A number of these women stated that they may not feel so welcome in other parts of the United States. In contrast, for women such as Margot, the heightened militarization of the border exacerbated insecurity. As Anessa's account demonstrates, the extended closure of the US-Mexico border during the pandemic generated a sense of precarity for those who lost their sense of connection with family members on the other side. The particularities of a place intersect with immigration-related concerns to generate precarity. Attention to the role of context in producing emotions can help explain patterns that may seem perplexing from an epidemiological standpoint. As previously discussed, often missing from explanations of the Latina Health Paradox is attention to how unique factors in particular locations may contribute to health outcomes. For example, the degree of inclusiveness towards immigrants in a community, state-level immigration enforcement policies, and the quality of social networks may play a role in how welcome or unwelcome individuals feel. These factors may influence bodily experiences. Some of these bodily effects may be apparent in epidemiological analyses, while others may be invisible. Tellingly, Anessa was very open with me about experiencing depression during her pregnancy, yet her medical records failed to register this ailment.

Corporeal Kinship Effects of Immigration

Marla's account shows how the precarious situations of loved ones can fundamentally affect a person's well-being. Efraín's deportation disrupted all aspects of her life, and she described the resulting stress as the cause of her high blood pressure. When they were together in El Paso, Efraín had a stable income as a welder, enabling Marla to focus on school. Immediately after the deportation, Marla and her son moved to Juárez so that the family could remain together. This is also when Marla decided to put her school on hold; she had yet to return at the time of our interview given her need to generate income. When her son was old enough to start school, Marla decided it was time for them to return to living in El Paso, visiting Efraín in Juárez every weekend. She also took a job at a fast-food chain, needing to support their separate household. She described the strain of the transition: "The help was gone. I had to do everything on my own. I had to work. I had to take care of my kid. So it was being a full-time parent, plus having to work because I need the money." Her son also struggled with the transition; "he was refusing to learn English so that he could go back" to be with his father.

To keep the family as united as possible, Marla took her son to Juárez whenever she could. The constant border crossing involved dealing with long wait times to return to the United States and scrutiny from Border Patrol. At the time of our interview, Marla reported that it normally took her one to one and a half hours to cross back to El Paso, although she would allow for three hours if she was on her way to work, in case she had any problems.[2] She explained, "They usually check me a lot because I always go so often. They're always asking, 'How come you go? How come you cross so many times? What were you doing?' Like they're always on top of me because of that, because I cross so much. I cross sometimes four times a week, and during the summer, it's basically every day. So, they ask like many, many questions, and they put me through the X-ray, so that takes even more time. So that's why I'm always having to be giving myself at least three hours before my shift."

Prior to Efraín's deportation, Marla was one of an estimated twenty-two million people living in US households with at least one undocumented family member. In Texas, approximately 10.3 percent of the population resides with an undocumented family member (Mathema 2017). These figures fail to account for the affective ties that people may have for family members living outside of the household. Within our survey data, 61 percent of participants reported having at least one immediate family member without US citizenship, and of those, 31 percent reported concerns over the immigration status of an immediate family member. The extent to which our survey participants had acutely felt the direct effects of immigration policy was also striking—19 percent reported having at least one immediate family member who had been deported or held in immigration custody. As Marla's narrative shows, immigration policies have widespread ripple effects for US citizens, emphasizing the importance of examining the role of kinship ties in producing health disparities. Marla's explanatory model linked the stress produced by Efraín's immigration status and ultimate deportation to her high blood pressure and other adverse birth outcomes.

While Marla described a direct connection between her husband's precarious situation and her own health, embodied vulnerabilities do not always follow a clear path. Aurelia, a second-generation immigrant, described more complex ways that concerns for family members shaped her health and the health of her baby. Both Aurelia's parents were immigrants, but only her mother was undocumented. Compounding her mother's vulnerability was abuse from Aurelia's father. Aurelia explained:

> She [my mother] was deported a lot of times while I was growing up. My dad and my mom would fight a lot, so every time they would fight, my mom would go back to Mexico, and she would drag us with her. Then a few weeks, maybe months later, she decided to come back. We would see her literally crossing the river, and us just watching everything. Like, I've walked with them, like crossed together. I've been in detention centers. Them [Border Patrol], they never knew I was American; if not, they would've taken me away from my parents, but we've been detained.

The fact that immigration authorities detained Aurelia alongside her mother exhibits one of the ways immigration laws may deny the rights of nonwhite US citizens by virtue of their relationship to noncitizens. Aurelia described such experiences as causing anger and anxiety, which contributed to depression throughout her life. As a teenager, she struggled with an eating disorder, which she attributed to her mental state. She believes her eating disorder caused her daughter to have low birth weight and developmental delays. She said, "Before I got pregnant with her, I was very skinny. I wasn't eating right, and it had to do with my depression, my anxiety." While Aurelia's explanatory model did not directly link immigration concerns and her daughter's low birth weight, it illustrated an indirect route through which family relationships created embodied health vulnerabilities. Most significantly, Aurelia described the emotional responses generated by her mother's undocumented status as contributing to several mental and physical health ailments she believed caused her daughter's health problems.

For those in cross-border families, the effects of border and immigration policies may go beyond immigration status. In particular, border policies related to the War on Drugs have contributed to violence in Mexico.[3] While narcoviolence is widespread in various parts of Mexico and shifts based on cartel competition, homicide rates are consistently higher in border cities as cartels fight to control the crossing of drugs (Campbell 2010). As a result, although Mexico's northern border states encompass only 17.6 percent of the national population, they are the location of nearly half of all drug-related murders in the country (Ríos 2014).

Tamara was born in the United States to a US-citizen father and Mexican mother, who was originally from Durango. Her mother moved to live with her own parents in Juárez after she separated from Tamara's father. Because her family members had citizenship in their respective countries of residence, Tamara did not express immigration-related concerns over family, and she easily crossed the border to visit her Mexican relatives. It was the widespread violence in Mexico that touched her family and was a source of profound trauma for her. We interviewed Tamara in 2018, less than a year after the birth of her sixth child. During her pregnancy, cartel members in Juárez raped, tortured, and murdered her brother. The autopsy showed twenty-five bullet wounds, five of which were on his face. She keeps a video of the murder scene on her cell phone, which she pulled out during the interview, showing his body with a black garbage bag over his head—a common narco signature. Tamara cited the trauma resulting from her brother's murder as causing her to go into labor early and the near death of her baby.[4]

For Tamara, this experience of trauma was a moment within a lifetime of adverse events, demonstrating the ways different sources of stress can serve as compounding vulnerabilities for bodily ills. She first became pregnant at sixteen years old and subsequently had four children from two different relationships, both of which became abusive. The abuse in the household contributed to Tamara losing custody of her first four children. In the second relationship, she had three additional pregnancies that she did not carry to term. She had two miscarriages, which she attributed to her partner's abuse, including punches to the stomach. The third pregnancy ended with an abortion. According to Tamara, her partner forced her to have the abortion. She described wanting to be pregnant, as being pregnant was a source of joy and she cherished nurturing a human inside of her.

Clearly, Tamara's life history included many challenging circumstances that could contribute to poor birth outcomes. Yet, in recounting her life history, it was the murder of her brother that she described as her greatest source of pain, and the only time she became emotional during the interview was while speaking of his murder. It was also the event that was central to her explanatory model of preterm birth. Tamara's focus on her brother's murder highlights the ways kinship ties across borders can serve as one source of embodied vulnerability. As her narrative suggests, attention to transnational ties may offer a better understanding of negative birth outcomes among US citizens and those with a secure immigration status. Given that a significant proportion of first- and second-generation immigrants to the United States maintain familial ties in countries with high levels of violence (Pérez-Armendáriz 2021), concerns over family members left behind may generate embodied vulnerabilities.

Tamara's, Aurelia's, and Marla's experiences illustrate how having immigrant family members, being in mixed-status relationships, and having cross-border familial ties may contribute to health vulnerabilities. Aurelia and Marla described the emotional toll of detention and deportation of family members as a contributing factor to bodily ills. The ripple effects of policies emphasize that a person's well-being is never only about their individual positionality, but their connections to others. Attending to the emotions produced when harm occurs to loved ones can show how individuals perceive the risks faced by others as contributing to their own ill health.

Embodied Histories of Immigration-Related Vulnerability

Many of the naturalized citizens and permanent residents we interviewed had a history of being undocumented. Additionally, there were US citizens who grew up with undocumented family members who at some point gained legal status. These women often described the period of being undocumented or having undocumented family members as marked by significant levels of fear and anxiety. For example, Julia became a naturalized citizen in 2016 at the age of twenty-eight. She gained permanent residency before that through marriage to a US citizen after being undocumented since she was seven. Although we spoke in English, which Julia described as her dominant language, she repeatedly used the Spanish word *impotente* (powerless) to describe her emotions related to being undocumented. She elaborated:

> I couldn't say it [that I was undocumented]. I always felt like it was something so private that I couldn't, you know. I remember in high school people would be like, "Let's go to Juárez. Let's go to thirsty Thursday," and I would be like, "Oh, I can't, like my mom's not going to let me." Like, having to lie about who I really was because you don't know how people are going to act or react to it, and I don't want to be judged. It was horrible because I feel like my whole life, it literally was a lie. Because nobody knew it. Everyone thought I was a citizen. It's literally, you're living in a lie because you can't be open about it.

Although Julia gained a sense of security after adjusting her status, she had decades of insecurity. Even after becoming a citizen, she had concerns over family members, especially her undocumented brother, reflecting the ways different types of immigration-related concerns and associated vulnerabilities can overlap.

Aída, who was forty-three years old at the time of our interview in 2018, also described a difficult past related to her undocumented status. Aída became a permanent resident when she was twenty-one, after being undocumented for a decade. She spent her teenage years and early adulthood working in the fields in New Mexico, receiving schooling only intermittently. She recalled one occasion when a workplace immigration raid resulted in her deportation: "I looked up, and a helicopter was above us. By the time we tried to run, it was too late." Since this occurred before the post-9/11 increased militarization of the border, Aída said she simply walked across the border two days after her deportation and returned to work.

Despite recalling stressful histories, neither Aída nor Julia linked their pasts to the pregnancy risks they experienced. Aída had high blood pressure and gestational diabetes during two of her eight pregnancies. Her fear of the implications of her conditions demonstrated an internalization of medicalized discourses of high-risk pregnancies common in both the United States and Mexico (Fleuriet and Sunil 2017). This medical discourse of risk fueled Aída's emotional distress during her most recent pregnancy. After describing the anxiety she felt, she said, "I believe the anxiety came from so much bad news over things that one has no control over. There is always so much bad news about death in childbirth. I thought that if my blood pressure went up or if I had diabetes again during pregnancy that it would give me preeclampsia and a stroke, and that would be it." Aída's mention of the news refers to widespread media coverage that Texas had the highest maternal mortality rate in the United States (MacDorman et al. 2016). Although subsequent research showed that problems with the state data collection system may have led to incorrect statistics on Texas's maternal mortality rate (MacDorman et al. 2018), this follow-up research received little coverage.

Julia was seven months pregnant during our interview in 2019. She described her pregnancy as healthy, although she had gestational diabetes during the pregnancy of her one-year-old son. She described the differences in the pregnancies in a way that evidenced she had internalized a common biomedical discourse about diabetes that prioritizes individual behaviors. However, she also linked her behaviors to her emotions. She said, "I ended up having gestational diabetes. It was just like my depression, where like I would eat bad. You know, I ended up messing up because coming from a family that has diabetes I should have taken care of myself more for the same reason. And I think it was my depression, my 'I don't care anymore' kind of feeling. I cared for my baby, but in a way, I guess I wasn't caring for my baby. Because I wasn't feeding him what he needed to be fed, you know?" In contrast, she described herself as happy during her second pregnancy, which she believed led to a healthier baby with fewer risks. Julia described the depression during her first pregnancy as primarily related to relationship problems with the father. Compounding these problems was the stress from sponsoring her parents' immigration petitions for an adjustment of status. Given the political climate, she worried her parents' applications could be rejected.

Salma's life history illustrates the ways kinship ties can produce historical traumas that have long-lasting health consequences. As discussed in the previous chapter, Salma's mother and older sister were both undocumented throughout Salma's childhood, although both had since been able to adjust their status. Salma described numerous adverse experiences as a child and young adult that she believed were in large part related to her mother's immigration status. Without an easy way to cross the border, Salma's mother often returned to Mexico for long periods of time until she could find a way to cross back. Salma would be left with her negligent stepfather, who surrounded the kids with drug addicts. Salma took it upon herself to care for her younger siblings. She said, "It was a lot of those gaps in my childhood where I was just left to figure it out. Like left at [age] four to cook your own ramen noodles and weenies and eggs because nobody's home. Like you just got to figure it out." Things got so bad that Salma left home in high school and sought a restraining order against her mother. However, her mother convinced her to return to the family. Salma explained:

> I turned fourteen going into ninth grade. My mom would still, you know, show up. We had an order of protection against her, but she would show up with the kids crying at the door. You know, "We miss you. The kids need you." So I had these sporadic times that I would just go and stay at her house to watch the kids, but it was the same old same old. My mom would vanish and I was stuck with the kids. I still had to get them ready for school. I mean, I would wake up at 4:00 [a.m.] to get them ready for school and feed them. I would show up at high school with black bags under my eyes, just a mess, but I was able to continue.

After graduating from high school, Salma quickly became pregnant and throughout her twenties became caught in an abusive relationship that she struggled to leave. The anxiety and depression generated by this situation led her into psychiatric institutions multiple times, where she finally found the support she needed to leave the relationship. Although Salma had turned her life around and had been in a healthy relationship for several years prior, she still felt the reverberations of her early life through various ills, especially her diagnosis of type 2 diabetes and her mental health struggles.

Salma made direct connections between past traumas and her current health status, although Aída and Julia did not emphasize these links. However, even when individuals do not explicitly note a history of stress in their explanatory models, it is important to consider how past experiences can translate into adverse health outcomes. Arline Geronimus (1992) proposes the idea of *weathering* to explain how the cumulative stress, such as that which characterized Salma's, Julia's, and Aída's early life, can generate a lifetime of vulnerability to adverse health conditions, especially during pregnancy and the postpartum period. Notably, Julia and Aída reported having gestational diabetes, and Salma had developed type 2 diabetes in her early thirties. Given that stress hormones can alter glycemic regulation, there is growing research on the ways adverse life events can contribute to the onset of diabetes and exacerbate its severity (Lloyd, Smith, and Weinger 2005). The idea of weathering helps explain how the stress of poverty, being a minority, having an insecure immigration situation, and other adverse life circumstances and structural constraints can translate into health disparities, even later in life among individuals who have escaped adverse conditions. Within social epidemiology, weathering is often linked to ascribed statuses, particularly racialized groups. As Aída's and Julia's narratives suggest, applying this concept to immigrant populations can help attend to the unevenness of weathering. Both women described years of heightened vigilance, yet they both felt relief after gaining legal status. In such circumstances, weathering is a dynamic and irregular process, where individuals may have chronic stress followed by periods of relief when conditions improve. Such an approach can account for the role of past experiences in fueling stress-sensitive conditions, even after a person's circumstances have improved.

Embodiment and the Production of Local Biologies

In the local biologies of the border, immigration policies are a crucial sociopolitical factor contributing to embodied health vulnerabilities. Inclusion or exclusion generated by policies has health implications (Mattes and Lang 2020). Women perceived the implementation of immigration policy as a significant source of emotional distress that was potentially harmful during pregnancy. Their narratives support what medical research suggests about the health consequences of the stress response. The embodiment of immigration policies may play a significant role in patterns of birth outcomes in the region, even for those with a secure immigration status.

Women's narratives also show the uneven effects of immigration policies as they interact with the many particularities of the border. For some women, especially those originally from the northern border region of Mexico, living in a border city had protective features. Some women with limited time in the United States expressed minimal fear of the consequences of deportation because deportation would not involve a significant geographical move. For these women, the border may have a mediating effect on exclusionary policies by fostering a sense of belonging due to shared language and cultural background. They may feel more welcomed, particularly as Mexican immigrants, compared to what immigrants in other geographic locations experience. For others, the militarization of the border exacerbated insecurities as the constant presence of immigration officials generated heightened vigilance that women described as negatively affecting their health. These differences in how place can shape an individual's emotions highlight the importance of attending to subjective experiences and locating them in specific places and sociopolitical moments.

Women's narratives also show the significance of the temporal dimensions of embodiment in producing local biologies. What was happening at a particular moment contributed to the degree that the immigration status of a woman and her loved ones generated emotional distress. Although the border has been heavily militarized for decades, women described additional anxieties resulting from the increased threats of detention and deportation occurring during the Trump administration. For women with a history of being undocumented, the political context they experienced in the past may be an important dimension to consider in relation to how their history of precarity might translate into health vulnerabilities.

Temporal considerations also bring attention to the differences between acute and chronic stress. Women's emotional distress in response to immigration-related concerns may include moments of acute crisis, as Marla described following the deportation of her husband. More common was the constant low-grade chronic anxiety resulting from the fear that such an event could occur. In many cases, women described conditions of chronic wariness punctuated by moments of more intense stress. Women suggested both types of stress had negative health implications. Tamara in particular described the acute stress following her brother's murder as the cause of her baby's preterm birth. Many women, in contrast, reflected on the toll of chronic stress resulting from the daily experience of having immigration-related concerns—an influence that was harder to pinpoint.

There is an inherent messiness to engaging with temporality. Our interlocutors shared several common immigration-related experiences, but what was going on politically and socially at a particular time in relation to their individual lives profoundly affected their emotional responses to these experiences. For example, Aída described her past deportation as not having a significant negative impact on her, since it occurred before the heightened militarization of the border, making it relatively easy for her to return. Marla, on the other hand, described how the deportation of her husband upended her life.

Immigration Policy as Reproductive Violence

As I conducted the research for this book, numerous epidemiological studies showed that restrictive immigration policies, immigration raids, and even threats of targeted enforcement are associated with adverse birth outcomes (Gutierrez and Dollar 2023; Krieger et al. 2018; Novak, Geronimus, and Martinez-Cardoso 2017; Torche and Sirois 2019). While these studies provide compelling statistical data, the women I interviewed did not need these statistics to tell them what they already knew all too well. Marla may wonder how the profound trauma of her husband's deportation while they had a newborn would *not* have negative consequences for her own health. As Margot narrates, it is the constant threat of deportation that has taken a toll on her health year after year. For these women, immigration policies enact reproductive violence by contributing to health vulnerabilities for themselves and their children. Beyond physical health risks, immigration policies also separate families, or threaten to separate them, limiting women's abilities to reproduce and raise children with dignity and security. While I have focused on the ways immigration and border policies factor into local biologies, the local biologies of the border are not only about the effects of border militarization. In the next chapter, I further engage with how a range of contextual factors of the border contribute to adverse health outcomes with a specific focus on preeclampsia.

3

The Local Biology of Preeclampsia

In November of 2020, Lupe entered the final weeks of her pregnancy. Seemingly out of the blue, dark spots began distorting her vision. Dark spots, flashes of light, and blurriness are among the visual disturbances people with preeclampsia commonly experience, possibly as a consequence of swelling in the brain or other irritations of the central nervous system. The nervous system is but one of the organ systems that may begin to fail as preeclampsia progresses. Lupe may also have been beginning to experience damage to her liver, kidney, and lungs. Symptoms of emerging organ dysfunction may vary and can include severe headache, pain under the ribs from an enlarged liver, visual disruptions, swelling of the face and hands, or even a vague sense of feeling unwell. In my own experience of developing preeclampsia, I had a sudden insatiable craving for sugar after having an aversion to sweets my entire pregnancy, possibly a result of my cells starving for energy that they could not readily access with my body in distress.

Preeclampsia can have a sudden onset with rapid progression. Lupe recalled, "It was just random. It's like one day I just didn't feel good, and the next day, I was like, 'Maybe I need to go to the hospital.'" When she arrived at the hospital, her blood pressure was 167 over 98, in contrast to the ideal reading of 115 over 70 she had at her first prenatal visit. This reading suggested she was nearing a hypertensive crisis. Without medical intervention, her blood pressure may have continued to rise, putting her in danger of a heart attack or stroke. Damage to the nervous system, indicated by Lupe's visual disturbances, could have also progressed, increasing the potential for a life-threatening seizure, which distinguishes the more severe diagnosis of eclampsia from preeclampsia. The word eclampsia comes from the Greek word for lightning, with the medical label likely originating from the frequent reports of flashes of light prior to an eclamptic seizure (Purkenson and Vekerdy 1999).[1]

Upon her admission to the hospital, Lupe's doctor informed her that they would induce labor. Induction of labor, alongside the administration of drugs to control dangerous symptoms such as high blood pressure, are the primary medical interventions for managing preeclampsia when it occurs in the final weeks of pregnancy. This is because the only cure for preeclampsia is delivery of the placenta. Preeclampsia likely occurs in some pregnant people due to the way the placenta implants in the uterine wall, with a shallow implantation possibly hampering the exchange of blood across the placenta between the pregnant person and fetus (Roberts and Gammill 2005). Delivery of the baby and placenta typically halts further organ damage. Early-onset preeclampsia is less common than preeclampsia during the final weeks of pregnancy but involves greater risks necessitating complicated decisions about balancing the increasing threat to the pregnant person's health and the adverse outcomes associated with inducing preterm delivery. Even with timely medical intervention, early-onset preeclampsia remains a leading cause of preterm birth, low birth weight, and neonatal mortality (Davies, Bell, and Bhattacharya 2016).

In the absence of medical interventions that facilitate the induction of labor and management of symptoms, preeclampsia is significantly more likely to escalate and result in more severe organ damage, a stroke, or an eclamptic seizure. Of those who develop eclampsia, one-third will likely die without timely intervention. Preeclampsia can also precede HELLP (hemolysis, elevated liver enzymes, and low platelets) syndrome, which can lead to life-threatening blood clots, pulmonary edema, kidney failure, or liver failure, or a combination of these symptoms. The high death rate associated with untreated preeclampsia and eclampsia make these conditions a leading cause of maternal death on a global scale, especially in resource-poor contexts with limited access to emergency obstetric interventions (Ghulmiyyah and Sibai 2012). In the United States, preeclampsia remains a primary contributing factor for maternal mortality and morbidity, suggesting that there are forces interrupting a timely diagnosis and optimal intervention (Shih et al. 2016).

Fortunately, Lupe recognized something was wrong, had coverage under Medicaid for Pregnant Women that eased her concerns about going to the emergency room, and received a prompt intervention that included inducing labor. After two days of labor, her cervix had not yet fully dilated. Her doctor informed her that there were indications of fetal distress and that they would be moving to a C-section. Delivery via an uncomplicated C-section may last less than twenty minutes. However, preeclampsia and medication used in the management of the condition increase the risk of hemorrhaging, which can complicate a C-section (Eskild and Vatten 2009).[2] Lupe began hemorrhaging and the surgery lasted over two hours.

Following the delivery, Lupe remained in the hospital for three days under treatment with magnesium sulfate to manage her blood pressure. As the father of the baby was no longer in Lupe's life, she had brought her mother as her birthing companion. Because the baby was born during the COVID-19 pandemic, COVID-19 restrictions meant that no one else could accompany her in the hospital, even when her mother had to leave to return to work. Lupe thus spent multiple days alone in her hospital room with her newborn. She felt overwhelmed and unable to properly care for her own bodily needs given the surgical trauma she had barely begun to recover from and lack of a support person. Lupe felt that the nursing staff could have been more helpful given that she was by herself with a newborn following a C-section. She felt further invalidated after asking one of her nurses what might have caused the preeclampsia. The nurse responded, "Sometimes that happens when a single mother has a baby."

Preeclampsia is a complex, poorly understood medical condition. It was not possible for the nurse to provide Lupe with a definitive answer as to why she developed preeclampsia. The nurse's explanation may have been an attempt to consider the ways social circumstances can function as social determinants of health. Yet, the lack of sensitivity in her comment reflects a broader pattern in biomedicine, which has a tendency to individualize risk, even when accounting for potential social determinants of health. This individualized approach is strikingly clear in the biomedical framing of risk for preeclampsia. The American College of Obstetrics and Gynecology's defining of risk factors for preeclampsia is telling. The list of risk factors includes primarily biological variables, such as maternal age, preexisting hypertension, diabetes, obesity, and renal disease. The list does also include sociodemographic factors, namely being African American and having low socioeconomic status (ACOG 2020). As Jasmin Johnson and Judette Louis (2022) point out, the inclusion of race and socioeconomic status attends to social vulnerabilities but often only at the individual level, failing to account for multilevel factors that produce risk. There is nothing inherently biological about a person's race or socioeconomic status that put them at increased risk; rather, systemic racism, health care exclusion, discrimination, structural violence, and environmental injustice produce a disproportionate burden of vulnerability for racialized and socially marginalized populations.

I use women's experiences of preeclampsia to push back against frameworks that individualize risk. The medical literature demonstrates that preeclampsia is a biosocial condition. In other words, while preeclampsia involves biological processes, it also involves bodily responses to social phenomena. The border context involves a set of social, political, and environmental conditions that may contribute to the high burden of preeclampsia among populations that have been subjected to acute and chronic social stress as well as greater potential exposure to environmental contamination. As noted earlier, there was a strikingly high rate of preeclampsia among participants in our 2020–22 study. Nearly 25 percent of survey participants (n = 176) had a preeclampsia diagnosis, compared to a national prevalence rate of 4 percent (Bibbins-Domingo et al. 2017). Various aspects of women's social lives may have factored into their vulnerability. Tellingly, the prevalence rate varied based on whether a woman had CHIP Perinatal or Medicaid, which to some extent serves as a proxy for immigration status. Women with CHIP Perinatal, who were much more likely to have a precarious immigration status, had a preeclampsia prevalence rate of 31 percent compared to a prevalence of 23 percent for women with Medicaid. There was also an association between reported levels of COVID-related stress and a preeclampsia diagnosis. Women who reported moderate to severe stress as a consequence of the pandemic had a 36 percent prevalence rate of preeclampsia, compared to a prevalence rate of 20 percent among women who reported a lower burden of stress caused by the pandemic. Interview narratives further elucidate how women's social worlds were central to the biological processes involved in preeclampsia as well as the cascade of risks that result from having this condition.

Preeclampsia as a Complex Biosocial Syndrome

James Roberts, a physician and one of the most prolific biomedical experts on preeclampsia, proposes that the condition has multiple etiologies (see Roberts and Gammill 2005). While abnormal placentation (implantation of the placenta) may be a root cause of preeclampsia, the syndrome manifests for only some people with the same abnormalities. In other words, placentation may predispose someone to preeclampsia, but subsequent development of the disease is not inevitable. Multiple maternal factors and physiological pathways can determine whether a person goes on to develop the condition. There are likely regional factors that can cause preeclampsia to manifest in distinct ways in different populations (Roberts and Bell 2013). To understand how and why local particularities are important, some understanding of the biosocial processes involved in preeclampsia is useful. Table 3.1 explains key biological factors involved in the progression of preeclampsia and how socioenvironmental conditions influence this biology.

What would lead to a preeclampsia prevalence rate of 24.9 percent among the 176 participants in our research?[3] As I began studying maternal health in El Paso, I often heard OB-GYNs (doctors of obstetrics and gynecology) and midwives comment on the high rate of preeclampsia in the region. Yet, having nearly one in four women receive this diagnosis initially seemed so stark a contrast to the national data that I at times questioned the validity of our findings. In further conversations with providers, those who cared primarily for a population similar to those captured in our research—Latinas using publicly funded care during the height of the pandemic—agreed that this figure aligned with their clinical experiences. However, the burden within the community is uneven, as the overall prevalence rate in El Paso is likely not as high as what we found in our sample. Due to a lack of data, it is impossible for me to say just how much the prevalence rate varies locally. Since hospitals are not required to report incidences of preeclampsia, many do not formally track it. The medical school that I collaborated with, for example, had no way of providing me with a prevalence rate among births at the associated teaching hospital given that they do not track cases. And while birth certificate data is an important source of data on births, preeclampsia is not among the variables recorded on birth certificates. Even

TABLE 3.1: Medical Terms Related to the Biosocial Progression of Preeclampsia

	Definition	Role in preeclampsia	Relationship with socioenvironmental factors
Oxidative stress	Condition in which the body is unable to remove toxins quickly enough to maintain homeostasis.	Abnormal placentation can lead to oxidative stress. When the body is experiencing oxidative stress, it is more prone to inflammatory conditions, diabetes, high blood pressure, and preeclampsia (Aouache et al. 2018).	Exposure to environmental pollution and the stress response can interfere with endocrine signaling involved in oxidative stress (Daiber and Münzel 2020).
Endothelial dysfunction	The endothelium is the inner lining of the heart and blood vessels and produces nitric oxide. A drop in nitric oxide production (endothelial dysfunction) causes arteries to narrow, which can result in high blood pressure.	May be caused by oxidative stress and other maternal inflammatory responses triggered by abnormal placentation. For a person with preexisting endothelial dysfunction, abnormal placentation may be more likely to lead to preeclampsia (Alexander 2007).	Frequency of exposure to and intensity of chronic stress contribute to endothelial dysfunction (Sher et al. 2020).
Systemic inflammation	An overstimulation of immune responses. This proinflammatory state can make a person vulnerable to many health ailments.	Can interfere with placentation, increasing predisposition to preeclampsia (Lee et al. 2012). Can exacerbate oxidative stress, making the development of preeclampsia more likely and/or more severe (Redman and Sargent 2004).	Social stress, chronic disease, and exposure to toxins can put the body in a proinflammatory state.

at the state level, it is difficult to find good data given that Texas does not have a perinatal data system. Some states collect data on preeclampsia as a part of the Pregnancy Risk Assessment Monitoring System (PRAMS). However, the Centers for Disease Control and Prevention (CDC) only releases raw data from states that achieve a minimum response rate on the survey. Texas has not achieved a high enough response rate since 2012, and the state did not collect data on preeclampsia at that time.[4]

There are some indications that Mexicans and Mexican Americans have a higher rate of preeclampsia than other groups. For example, Jian Gong and colleagues (2012) examined preeclampsia rates by national origin for births in New York City from 1995–2003. While Latinas as a whole had a prevalence rate similar to that of white women, when broken down by nationality, Mexican-origin women were 2.5 times more likely to have preeclampsia than white women. Still, the overall preeclampsia prevalence rate among Mexican-origin women in this study was 5 percent,[5] suggesting that geographic disparities may be one factor contributing to the even higher rate in El Paso. This regional burden is likely not limited to the US side of the border. Although public health reporting systems in Mexico maintain poor records of preeclampsia, Prudencia Cerón-Mireles (2006) found that the rate of maternal mortality from preeclampsia is significantly higher along Mexico's northern border in comparison to other parts of the country, despite the higher level of economic development in this region.

While contextual factors are likely a key factor in the preeclampsia rate at the regional level, the additional vulnerabilities faced by a marginalized subpopulation during the COVID-19 pandemic may have compounded this disease burden, producing the startling prevalence rate we found. A life in a toxic environment, the cumulative stress associated with one's social position, and a lifetime of limited access to care are but a few of the vulnerabilities that characterized the lives of women we interviewed and reflect patterns that are prevalent among marginalized populations in the region. To dissect how contextual factors and social inequities likely contribute to the cascade of events involved in the development of preeclampsia, it is useful to return to the concept of local biologies.

Local Biologies and Syndemic Interactions in the Border Context

Local biologies attends to the entanglement of social and biological processes (Lock 2017). The characteristics of a given place—the presence of environmental toxins, a legacy of historical injustices, and the execution of policies, among other social forces—can produce biological differences and shape the social experience of a condition (Brotherton and Nguyen 2013; Moran-Thomas 2019). Further, there is a need to consider temporality and how conditions may manifest in different ways in relation to what is happening. While the particularities of a place at a given moment are a key concern, this context may carry distinct meanings and set the stage for different experiences for a person based on their social position and other individual-level factors.

Some regional patterns in the manifestation of preeclampsia may involve what Merrill Singer (2009) describes as *syndemic interactions*. The term *syndemic* brings attention to the synergistic effect of multiple conditions. In other words, the presence of one condition can exacerbate the effects of other conditions that are present. The root word synergy emphasizes that the resulting health consequences may be greater than simply the sum of each individual condition. According to Singer, the ways that diseases may interact go beyond disease pathology, as factors in the social and environmental context contribute to how pathogens progress and feed off each other. In the border context at the height of the COVID-19 pandemic, it appears that preeclampsia, diabetes,[6] emotional distress, and the COVID-19 virus may have involved syndemic interactions.

Substantial research shows that the US-Mexico border region has disproportionately high rates of obesity, hypertension, and diabetes (Fisher-Hoch et al. 2010; Vijayaraghavan et al. 2010), which have potentially synergistic relationships with preeclampsia as well as other health conditions. As such, these diseases carry the label of "underlying conditions." The term *underlying condition* carries substantial explanatory weight in medical discourse, even though it fails to address what causes disease interactions and instead furbishes a weak explanation for morbidity and mortality rates. For example, public health officials explained away the high burden of severe COVID-19 infections and deaths in the region as a consequence of underlying conditions. But where does the risk of underlying conditions originate? Despite medical discourses that continue to emphasize the role of behaviors, especially diet and exercise, it is becoming increasingly clear that these individual variables are only a small piece of the complex array of factors that contribute to underlying conditions. As Abril Saldaña-Tejeda (2021) argues, the individualization of underlying conditions that contributed to COVID-19 deaths detracted attention away from the underlying conditions of poverty, state neglect, racism, and structural violence.

A toxicology paradigm for approaching disease etiology moves the focus from the individual to the environment. This paradigm shows how the explosion of toxins in the environment as a characteristic of a capitalist world system generates vulnerability to an array of diseases, including the underlying conditions that increase the likelihood of

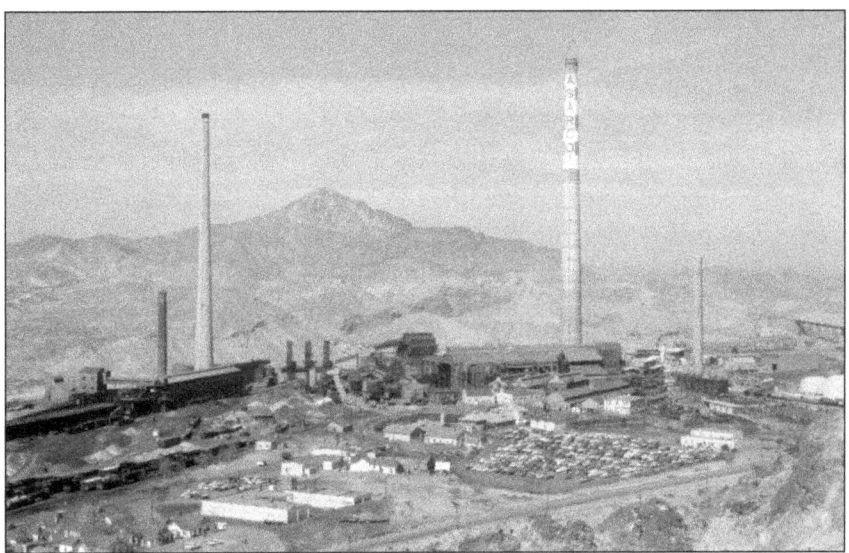

Figure 3.1: ASARCO's "Smeltertown" in 1975
Credit: Courtesy University of Texas at El Paso Library Special Collections Department, historical records of the former ASARCO smelter site, M5585

developing preeclampsia (Neel and Sargis 2011). Significant to El Paso is a legacy of environmental injustice that has led to persistently high levels of air, water, and soil pollution (Hampton and Ontiveros 2019; Uribarri 2021) and the city ranking as one of the most polluted cities in the United States (American Lung Association 2021). The historical legacy of environmental injustice includes the 1887–1999 operation of a heavy metal smelter in El Paso operated by American Smelting and Refining Company (ASARCO) beginning in 1901. The plant became notorious after blood samples from area school children showed lead levels four times higher than acceptable limits. Recent analyses of soil samples from neighborhoods adjacent to the now closed plant show persistent high concentrations of heavy metals, especially lead but also cadmium (Robinson 2017). There is strong evidence pointing to a link between elevated maternal cadmium levels and preeclampsia (for a review, see Rosen et al. 2018).

More recently, a number of border industrialization policies have had negative implications for the local environment. For example, the maquiladora industry[7] exploded following the passage of the North American Free Trade Agreement (NAFTA) in 1994; in the subsequent five years, 1,450 new plants opened in Mexico's northern border region (Gereffi 2018). The maquiladora industry produces high levels of air, soil, and water pollution, and there are profound health effects resulting from this contamination (Grineski and Juárez-Carrillo 2012). Although these plants are on the Mexican side of the border, weather patterns result in environmental contamination on both sides. Further, long wait times to cross international bridges contribute to air pollution throughout the region. During peak crossing hours, it is normal to wait hours to cross into the United States. When crossing in a vehicle, this is time spent with an idling engine.[8] As a consequence of these various patterns, air samples from the region show that air pollutants frequently exceed air quality standards (Li et al. 2011). Exposure to nitrogen dioxide, which occurs through proximity to dense traffic, likely increases the risk for developing preeclampsia (Rosen et al. 2018). Nitrogen dioxide is also among the toxic chemicals produced from oil refineries. A major oil refinery lies only three miles from downtown El Paso, possibly exacerbating preeclampsia risks for the residents in the densely populated vicinity. The extreme heat of summer months may further amplify the risks produced by air pollution, especially when the pregnant person experiences greater heat exposure in the first or third trimester (Shashar et al. 2020).

The environmental toxins prevalent in the border region include endocrine disrupting chemicals that alter hormone signaling and endocrine functioning in ways that potentially increase the likelihood of developing multiple metabolic disorders, especially diabetes and obesity. As such, some scholars alternatively refer to these chemicals as *obesogens*. Several studies have documented an association between exposure to endocrine disrupting chemicals and preeclampsia (Bearblock, Aiken, and Burton 2021; Lee et al. 2012; Malmqvist et al. 2013). The full extent that environmental toxins may contribute to preeclampsia is still unknown given the lack of research on the role of specific chemicals (Rosen et al. 2018).

Beyond the physical environment, shared experiences of social disadvantage may also contribute to the high prevalence of preeclampsia. Emotional responses to social experiences may play an important mediating role. Researchers have found that a number of measures of emotional distress have a positive association with preeclampsia. There is an especially strong link between a person's lifetime history of anxiety or depression and development of preeclampsia (Zhang et al. 2013). Further, there is evidence that it is not just mental health status alone, but also how mental health relates to other conditions, that exacerbates risk. Yunxian Yu and colleagues (2013) found that a high burden of psychosocial stress combined with preexisting hypertension (which is already stress sensitive) can increase the likelihood a person will develop preeclampsia by twenty times. At the physiological level, emotional distress activates inflammatory responses, producing a number of hormones that can have deleterious effects, especially when stress is chronic.[9] Cortisol, a key stress hormone, may play a role in how the social context contributes to vulnerability to preeclampsia. In our analysis of hair samples, we found a higher median cortisol concentration in hair samples from women who developed preeclampsia compared to those who did not develop the disease (see appendix I for further discussion). As we have seen, the widespread emotional distress produced by immigration and border policies has ripple effects throughout the region, but it may have especially profound effects for those who are undocumented, have undocumented family members, have binational families, or have a history of being undocumented.

Temporality is also an important dimension of the local biology of preeclampsia, especially considering we conducted research during the first two years of the COVID-19 pandemic. Early in the COVID-19 pandemic, it became clear that patients who tested positive for COVID-19 during pregnancy were also significantly more likely to develop preeclampsia (Papageorghiou et al. 2021).[10] Further research has clarified that COVID-19 infection can increase the likelihood a person will develop preeclampsia in multiple ways. The timing of COVID-19 infection during pregnancy is significant. If COVID-19 infection occurs during the first trimester, while the placenta is still forming, the inflammatory state produced by COVID-19 infection can contribute to abnormalities in placentation. As a result, COVID-19 infection during the first trimester may predispose a person to preeclampsia as well as other placental problems (Rad et al. 2022).[11] When COVID-19 infection occurs later in pregnancy, it can create a proinflammatory state, even when a person is asymptomatic. This predisposes a person to not only developing preeclampsia but having more severe effects of the condition (Coronado-Arroyo et al. 2021). The dangers of severe preeclampsia are especially high if COVID-19 infection occurs in the final week of pregnancy (Papageorghiou et al. 2021).[12]

Experiential Manifestations of Preeclampsia

The narratives of four women, Sandra, Janeth, Lina, and Lupe, reflect different ways the local landscape and individual positionalities contribute to vulnerabilities for developing preeclampsia and the lived experience of the condition. For Sandra and Janeth, diabetes and the COVID-19 pandemic factored into their vulnerabilities, but in different ways. Janeth's and Lina's narratives highlight the role of emotional distress and how their social lives produced this distress. Lupe's experiences show how postpartum preeclampsia poses even greater hazards to a person's health. Situating these women's narratives within the contours of the border region highlights the significance of time and place in producing their vulnerabilities and shaping their experiences. It is these contextual factors that are often absent from approaches that individualize risk.

Sandra: Preeclampsia, Diabetes, and COVID-19

In November of 2020, El Paso was quickly becoming ground zero for COVID-19 deaths in the United States. That month marked the first time that the State of Texas deployed the National Guard to the county to assist with managing the corpses from COVID-19 deaths. Prior to that, inmates had been handling the bodies (Samuels 2020). By the end of the month, the El Paso Convention Center served as a field hospital. Having run out of mobile morgues to store the dead, the county opened a refrigerated warehouse for this purpose (Willard 2020). The city monitoring system showed an average of over one thousand new cases per day during the first two weeks of November 2020 (El Paso Strong 2020). Given the hours-long wait times at testing sites and the absence of home testing, it is likely that positive cases were much higher than the official statistics.

It was within this context of a public health disaster that Sandra gave birth to her third child when she was thirty-three years old. Given her history of diabetes, which included gestational diabetes during her first pregnancy and a subsequent diagnosis of type 2 diabetes at the age of twenty-four, her doctor recommended induction at thirty-seven weeks' gestation. Since a pregnant person with diabetes is at greater risk of pregnancy and birth complications, providers often encourage induction for a person with any type of diabetes once the pregnancy reaches full-term.[13]

The week prior to Sandra's planned induction, her mother tested positive for COVID-19. Sandra began developing symptoms shortly after and feared how her own possible COVID-19 infection would affect the baby and the birth. After testing positive, Sandra's provider recommended that they delay the planned induction until she recovered, to prevent transmission of the virus to her newborn. Her induction was rescheduled for thirty-eight weeks' gestation. In the meantime, the baby turned into a breech position and Sandra developed preeclampsia. This combination of factors led to a C-section.

The trifecta of conditions experienced by Sandra—diabetes, COVID-19, and preeclampsia—may have emerged in tandem due to their synergistic interactions. Preeclampsia and diabetes present as distinct diseases, with no overlapping diagnostic criteria. Yet, there is a strong correlation between preeclampsia and diabetes; a person who may be predisposed to preeclampsia due to abnormal placentation is more likely to go on to develop symptoms of preeclampsia if they also have diabetes (McElwain et al. 2020). Both conditions make a person more vulnerable to cardiovascular complications later in life. Further, gestational diabetes can alter glucose metabolism, increasing the likelihood that a person with gestational diabetes will later develop type 2 diabetes (Shen et al. 2018), as was the case for Sandra following her first pregnancy. For Sandra, having type 2 diabetes during subsequent pregnancies significantly increased her risk for preeclampsia, highlighting the importance of a person's health through their life course for understanding the implications of disease interactions.

Sandra's body mass index (BMI) fell into the obese range, which also factored into her vulnerability for developing diabetes and preeclampsia

(Roberts et al. 2011). Diabetes and obesity are often explained away as a consequence of individual behaviors, especially diet and exercise, despite mounting evidence showing how metabolic disorders may be a consequence of the complex interplay between the environment, social stress, epigenetic factors, historical traumas, and individual dispositions (Moran-Thomas 2019).

Sandra's narrative shows the ways her social position generated vulnerabilities and affected her experiences of her conditions. Sandra described herself as a Dreamer, meaning she spent her childhood and early adulthood undocumented after her parents relocated the family from Juárez when she was seven years old. Having protection under Deferred Action for Childhood Arrivals (DACA) since 2012 gave her a sense of security she did not previously have, including an ability to legally seek employment. This stability, however, remained contingent upon political actions. She was grateful she was able to renew her DACA status prior to Donald Trump taking presidential office and she expressed hope that Joe Biden would pass immigration reform. Despite this limited sense of security regarding her own immigration status, she still had many family members, including her husband, who were undocumented. Their precarious status posed limitations on the benefits their household could receive, and such support could have helped offset the challenges they faced during the pandemic. Most importantly, early in her pregnancy, both Sandra and her husband lost their jobs, leading to economic struggles and food insecurity. Sandra qualified for unemployment, but her husband did not because he worked in the informal economic sector. It took months for her husband to find a new job. Sandra also received the COVID-19 stimulus checks given that her DACA status allowed her to have a social security number, but her husband's undocumented status prevented him from receiving the checks. The resulting economic stress limited Sandra's ability to have a healthy diet, and her feelings of emotional distress possibly contributed to physiological risks. Chronic stress can cause persistent surges in glucose, and chronically elevated glucose levels increase diabetes risk. The stress response also produces cortisol, a hormone that cues fat storage and stimulates cravings for sugar. Cumulative stress throughout Sandra's life course, in part from her previous undocumented status, may have contributed to her higher BMI and vulnerability for developing diabetes.

COVID-19 infection likely further compounded Sandra's risk for developing preeclampsia. However, her primary concern was how her positive test result shaped how hospital personnel treated her when it was time to deliver. Although Sandra and her husband had their release from isolation letters from the city's public health department, she had to fight in order for her husband to accompany her during the birth. She explained:

> They were still giving me a hard time and telling me that, no my husband was not gonna be there. I'm like, "Yes, my husband is gonna be with me, I have a letter, a clearance letter from the health department and he's gonna be with me. You could call whoever you want." I gave them a hard time, and yeah, sure enough they let us up. But as soon as we went up to labor and delivery, they gave me a hard time there too. The lady told me, "I need to talk to my supervisor," and I'm like, "Talk to whoever you want, but my husband is gonna be with me during delivery." I was getting anxious. I'm like, I'm not gonna have my baby without my husband being with me.

Following the birth, the pandemic continued to put pressure on Sandra and her household. When I interviewed her eight months postpartum, she had still not returned to work. With her children needing to be home for virtual schooling and the health of her newborn at stake, she decided it would be better to stay at home until the public health situation improved. Fortunately, she was able to receive extended unemployment benefits following passage of the American Rescue Plan, which made it financially possible for her to care for her children and avoid additional risks to her newborn's health. However, the challenges of not having childcare during extended school closures had made it difficult for Sandra to manage her diabetes postpartum. While her CHIP Perinatal coverage had long ended, she did qualify for the public hospital's discount program, which enabled her to seek care for a cost she described as affordable. Such charity programs vary dramatically by hospital system and are most often available through county public hospitals. In this sense, while contextual factors contributed to her health risks, it was local public health policies that afforded some protections when care would otherwise be out of reach as a consequence of state- and national-level policies.

Janeth: The Pandemic, Mental Health, and Preeclampsia

Like Sandra, Janeth's dual diagnosis of gestational diabetes and preeclampsia complicated her third pregnancy. The COVID-19 pandemic also significantly impacted her health, even though, at the time of our interview, she had never tested positive for COVID-19. Rather, it was the mental health burden generated by the pandemic causing her ill health. She explained, "I did get very, very depressed during the pregnancy. I had my husband and other two girls to be with me to help me through it. Also, my husband became unemployed and it was just a very, very, very stressful pregnancy. I was at risk, I want to say, because I was having suicidal thoughts during the pregnancy."

Although Janeth described some mental health struggles in her previous two pregnancies, she felt that her most recent pregnancy was distinct. She went on to attribute her mental health status to her fears of the virus and the economic struggles her family experienced as a consequence of her husband losing his job during the pandemic. Prior to these pandemic struggles, she was already mourning that immigration policies had torn her family apart. Just before the pandemic, her aunt's, uncle's, and grandfather's asylum claims were denied, leading to their deportations to Mexico. This experience created profound sadness for Janeth, especially when her grandfather passed away during the pandemic and she was unable to attend his funeral.

Given that Janeth had coverage under Medicaid for Pregnant Women, she was able to access health care beyond her prenatal visits and received a referral to a psychiatrist. Her treatment included taking antidepressants and anti-anxiety medication during the pregnancy. Following a diagnosis of gestational diabetes in the second trimester, her provider also recommended that she begin taking baby aspirin to reduce the risk of developing preeclampsia. Despite this preventive measure and having blood pressure readings consistently in the lower end of the normal range until the final weeks of pregnancy, Janeth developed preeclampsia. As a result, her provider induced labor at thirty-seven weeks' gestation. The baby weighed 2,449 grams, just below the cutoff of what is considered to be a low birth weight, which is 2,500 grams. While thirty-seven weeks is full-term, the low birth weight is an indication that the baby's health could have benefitted from additional time in the womb if Janeth had not developed preeclampsia.

Postpartum, Janeth continued to struggle with the mental health consequences of the pandemic and hesitated to go to doctor's visits due to potential exposure to COVID-19. When she began experiencing what she knew was likely postpartum depression, she feared what she might do to her baby and called her doctor. Her doctor was available that day for a telehealth visit, and she quickly received a referral to a therapist. Her continued Medicaid coverage during the public health emergency meant she was able to continue with her therapy for an extended period of time following the birth. Given her history of suicidal ideation, this may have been life-saving care for her.

Janeth's narrative suggests that the syndemic interactions generated by the COVID-19 pandemic were not just about COVID-19 infection. For her, the pandemic fueled significant mental health concerns, including suicidal thoughts. The medical research indicates that these emotions activate physiological responses that are significant for exacerbating risks for preeclampsia. Janeth's social position is important for understanding the extent of her pandemic-related distress. Given her family's already vulnerable socioeconomic situation, they acutely felt the effects of her husband's job loss. While they had been able to make ends meet through unemployment benefits and stimulus checks, Janeth continued to have anxiety over the possibility that they would not have enough money to pay their bills and feed their growing family. Even though Janeth and her husband were both US citizens, Janeth's extended family lacked such protections, contributing to her feeling that she should not ask family members for help if their situation became even more distressing.

Lina: Preeclampsia and Embodied Traumas

Between thirty-three and thirty-four weeks' gestation, Lina began having what felt like hot flashes. She said, "I would start to feel anxiety. Like just very hot." When she went for her thirty-four-week prenatal visit, her blood pressure was slightly elevated. Subsequent lab work indicated she may be developing preeclampsia, so her doctor ordered more frequent office visits for closer monitoring. In the subsequent weeks, her symptoms worsened, and her doctor scheduled her for induction as soon as she reached full-term at thirty-seven weeks' gestation. Of her preeclampsia diagnosis, Lina said, "It's because the stress was seriously just eating me inside."

In my first interview with Lina in the summer of 2021, she was at the beginning of the third trimester of a pregnancy that involved a "roller-coaster of emotions." Four days after her wedding, she found out she was pregnant. She had recently secured her dream job as an occupational therapist assistant and, before having a child, had wanted to work longer, save money, and buy a house with her husband, since they were living with family in San Antonio. Although they had not planned the pregnancy, her and her husband welcomed the news. However, following her twenty-week ultrasound, Lina faced what she described as the hardest decision of her life. The ultrasound showed that the fetus had fluid in the brain.

Weeks later, the fetus was diagnosed with meningocele, a mild form of spina bifida that involves little or no nerve damage. Although it is a neural tube defect, following surgery, any resulting disabilities are typically minor and treatable with therapy. However, at the time of her ultrasound, Lina did not receive a clear diagnosis, and instead, she described a traumatizing encounter with her doctor in San Antonio. She said, "I'm sorry, but he was an asshole about it. He was just so cold. Because of COVID, he didn't let my husband in so it was just me and him [the doctor] in a dark room. He was like, 'Indeed the baby has problems. See, it has a problem on the neck and then also it has liquid on the brain, so we're talking about severe mental retardation. He's probably never gonna walk, never gonna to talk. What do you want to do? Are you going to terminate the pregnancy?'"

Lina did in fact initially plan to terminate the pregnancy, and her husband and family supported her in this decision. When she decided that she could not go through with an abortion, in part because she felt like the pregnancy was part of God's plan for her, she continued to feel supported by her family. In continuing with the pregnancy, she and her husband decided to move back to El Paso to live with Lina's parents to have their help with the baby. In making this move, Lina and her husband gave up their jobs and lost their health insurance. As a US-born citizen,

Lina qualified for Medicaid to cover her prenatal care. Although she felt that she had made the right decision, she continued to question herself during the pregnancy. At one point she said, "Because of my faith, I am convinced I've made the right decision, but I don't know if I'm equipped to emotionally do it. Sometimes I doubt myself emotionally."

Not only did Lina implicate her stress levels as the cause of her preeclampsia, but she also described past traumas as the cause of her baby's spina bifida. The medical literature suggests that environmental toxins, diabetes, high fever early in pregnancy (e.g., from a COVID-19 infection), and a lack of maternal folic acid may be causes of spina bifida. Yet, when I asked Lina what she thought caused the condition, she said:

> You're going to think I'm crazy. I read this book called *It Didn't Start with You*. It talks about how trauma is passed on through generations. So when I read that book, it really resonated with me. I was like, okay, well this is really interesting 'cause you do see patterns in races. And so when I got pregnant and found out the problems with the baby, I started digging deeper into that. My head was like, "No, it couldn't just happen. There has to be a reason why." And so I started digging into that, into how trauma can really effect the future generations. If physically doctors cannot give me a diagnosis, at least I have this approach that is giving me the answer that I'm looking for and it helps.

Lina's narrative reflects one way of understanding the embodiment of historical traumas. It inherently made sense to her, as a racialized minority, that historical traumas could manifest as racial disparities in health. Interestingly, there is also substantial medical evidence that social and environmental issues, which have a burden more heavily felt by racialized minorities, can contribute to spina bifida. None of her providers equipped her with these explanations, instead telling her they did not know what caused the condition. Significantly, following a cluster of neural tube defects in the border city of Brownsville, Texas, the Texas Neural Tube Defect Project found that Texas-Mexico border residents have a higher rate of exposure to an array of factors that contribute to neural tube defects. Exposure to environmental toxins and nutritional deficiencies are particularly profound, especially in a person who has diabetes (Suarez et al. 2012). Researchers on this project also found that occupational exposure to chemical agents for health care workers heightened risks (Brender et al. 2002), an important dimension given Lina's employment in the health sector. Of additional significance is the fact that rates of neural tube defects on the Texas border are much higher than other parts of the United States, but they are similar to rates in Mexico (Suarez et al. 2012). While Lina was born in the United States, she spent most of her childhood living in Juárez, which has high rates of pollutants from the maquiladora industry (Grineski and Juárez-Carrillo 2012). She also crossed the US-Mexico border daily for school throughout her childhood, putting her in close contact with the air pollution produced from cross-border traffic delays.

Without this information offered to her, Lina searched for answers on her own. Her resulting explanatory model implicated past traumas for her son's condition. His uncertain diagnosis generated a burden of stress that she believes caused her to develop preeclampsia.

Lupe: Postpartum Preeclampsia as Compounding Vulnerabilities

Lupe developed preeclampsia in the final weeks of an otherwise healthy pregnancy. As we saw, preeclampsia contributed to a complicated birth that resulted in a C-section, for which she felt inadequately supported during her hospital stay. Lupe felt temporary relief when she returned home and had help from family members. A week later, however, she knew something was wrong. She feared returning to the hospital, since she would have to go alone. COVID-19 restrictions allowed one visitor while in labor and delivery, but no visitors for a return visit. She finally agreed to leave her newborn with her mother and the hospital admitted her for another three-day stay as her blood pressure remained at a dangerous level.

The return visit provided treatment for postpartum preeclampsia, but the ripple effects associated with this diagnosis lingered. She had already been struggling with getting her baby to latch to breastfeed. When she returned home from the hospital after her follow-up stay, her baby had become accustomed to a bottle and would not latch at all. Lupe tried pumping but became frustrated with how little milk she was able to extract with a breast pump. Worried she was starving her baby, she switched to formula. She expressed a sadness over what she felt like was a failure to provide for her baby, saying, "I thought something was wrong with me." Creating further challenges for her was the fact that the combination of preeclampsia and having major surgery meant that she was physically unable to return to work as quickly as her boss demanded. Lupe had requested two months of leave to recover and care for the baby. Her employer told her that she could have two months, but not the specific two months immediately after the birth. Given that she had been working at that job for less than twelve months, she did not yet have eligibility for leave under the Family and Medical Leave Act (FMLA). This detail legally enabled her employer to terminate her for being unable to return to work in the unreasonable timeframe they demanded.

Postpartum preeclampsia likely carries a higher risk of maternal morbidity and mortality than preeclampsia during pregnancy or at the time of birth. However, given poor reporting of postpartum preeclampsia, it is challenging to document the rate of complications associated with this condition (Hauspurg and Jeyabalan 2022). There are a number of reasons to suspect that postpartum preeclampsia poses particular dangers. For one, a significant percent of cases of postpartum preeclampsia present in individuals who showed no symptoms of preeclampsia until at least forty-eight hours after delivery. By this time, most people with an uncomplicated delivery have returned home. In one analysis of postpartum return visits to the emergency department, Lynne Yancey and colleagues (2011) found that over half of individuals diagnosed with postpartum preeclampsia had no previous diagnosis of the condition. Latinas and patients with a previous diagnosis of gestational diabetes are among the groups at greater risk of developing postpartum preeclampsia, without a prior diagnosis (Bigelow et al. 2014).[14] Given that symptoms of preeclampsia typically resolve following delivery, providers are often less on alert for postpartum preeclampsia and may be more likely to overlook concerns presented by a postpartum patient. This may be especially true if the person seeks care from a provider other than their midwife or OB-GYN (Hauspurg and Jeyabalan 2022).

As Lupe's experience shows, even with an earlier preeclampsia diagnosis, postpartum preeclampsia carried additional risks. While she had coverage for her return visit, she still faced significant challenges for even seeking care. Lupe was hesitant to return to the hospital in large part because it meant separation from her newborn. As a single mother, she could not rely on a partner to care for her baby. Fortunately, she had family members who could help, but many people lack this support network. COVID-era hospital policies that prohibited visitors exacerbated Lupe's concerns over separation from her baby. No one would even be able to bring her baby to visit or breastfeed during her hospital stay. Lupe had Medicaid for Pregnant Women, which ensured coverage for whatever care she received. For other women, financial concerns presented another barrier to seeking follow-up care. As we saw in the introduction, CHIP Perinatal did not cover Brisa's return visit to the hospital for postpartum preeclampsia. Given the severity of her condition, she was admitted to the public hospital and Emergency Medicaid could reimburse costs. Had the provider caring for Brisa not deemed her condition life-threatening, the hospital could have turned her away or presented her with a bill for thousands of dollars.

Rethinking Preeclampsia Risk

There is a tendency to attribute the high regional prevalence of preeclampsia to preexisting conditions, especially obesity, diabetes, and high blood pressure. There is some credibility to this explanation. As Sandra's medical history indicates, diabetes and obesity did increase her risk for developing preeclampsia. Gestational diabetes put Janeth at increased risk for preeclampsia, but this was not a preexisting condition prior to pregnancy. Lupe also had a BMI in the obese range, yet she did not have diabetes. None of these women's medical records or self-reports of health indicated a history of hypertension.

Attention to syndemic interactions elucidates the physiological processes that generate this increased disease burden. However, attributing the high prevalence of preeclampsia to preexisting conditions offers only a partial explanation. It fails to consider the contextual factors that have made people vulnerable to ill health in the first place—a life in a toxic environment, cumulative stress associated with one's social position, and a lifetime of limited access to care are but a few of the vulnerabilities that are prevalent in the region. While some individual providers are alert to these vulnerabilities, the biomedical framing of preeclampsia as a whole often lacks attention to the ways social forces produce individual risk.

Further, even when providers do recognize these social vulnerabilities, they only have the capacity to treat the health condition, rather than the social and environmental factors contributing to health vulnerabilities.

Laury Oaks and Barbara Herr Harthorn (2003) state that social difference and inequities factor into the development of health risk discourses. These discourses can then sustain the systems that produce health inequity. Individualizing risks such as obesity places the blame on individuals, failing to correct the social, political, and historical failures that contribute to ill health. Immigrant and minority women may experience added burdens of mother blame resulting from medical discourses that stigmatize cultural practices and traditional foods as unhealthy, while tasking women with changing their behaviors for the good of their families (Gálvez 2019). The medically prescribed individualized remedies for managing risk may at times be counterproductive. Although medical research identifies obesity as a risk factor, as Abril Saldaña-Tejeda (2021) argues, there is a need to rethink the production of this risk. Individualizing obesity as a risk factor can exacerbate stigma and detract attention from the social inequities that characterize everyday life of groups disproportionately burdened by obesity.

A lack of attention to social context detracts attention from many of the factors that contribute to risk for preeclampsia. Brisa's narrative illustrates the social vulnerabilities she felt due to her immigration status and economic marginalization. Her description of how these social vulnerabilities manifested as bodily experience aligns with medical research that shows how stress may produce physiological disruptions that increase the likelihood a person will develop preeclampsia. Brisa's medical records could be read as indications of a healthy patient, with a healthy BMI and ideal blood pressure at her first visit. Yet, attention to her social experiences reveal she did in fact have significant vulnerabilities. Some providers may be more attuned to these vulnerabilities than others. For example, providers within the practice where Brisa sought care often assume that patients with CHIP Perinatal are at greater risk, given their experiences caring for this population. However, even when providers recognize the social roots of preeclampsia, they are limited to the act of providing individual care.

The narratives presented in this chapter also suggest the importance of temporality in producing risk. The particularities of a given moment in time may exacerbate health vulnerabilities. For Sandra, COVID-19 infection may have played an important role in the fact that she developed preeclampsia. Janeth's description of how the pandemic affected her emotional well-being shows the embodied vulnerabilities generated by the social and economic effects of the pandemic. For women with immigration concerns, the execution of border and immigration policies during a particular period may be another factor that manifests as bodily harm.

Attention to the social context of risk for preeclampsia, and how individual experience within this context is contingent upon place, time, and a person's own positionality, is of particular importance for preeclampsia because of how quickly the condition may progress. Of note is the fact that a substantial portion (20–38 percent) of people in the United States who develop eclampsia did not have the common clinical indicators of hypertension or proteinuria prior to an eclamptic seizure (ACOG 2020). Closer monitoring of those who may be most vulnerable can help ensure a timely diagnosis to reduce the likelihood of maternal mortality and morbidity.[15]

Preeclampsia as a Symptom of Reproductive Violence

Individual experiences show how the particularities of the border region can manifest as reproductive harm, with preeclampsia and the social experience that it entails reflecting one of the pathways through which this harm occurs. Economic policies aimed at border industrialization and promoting commerce have contributed to environmental conditions that may alter the bodily physiology of local residents in ways that make a person more vulnerable to preeclampsia. Interventions that individualize resulting health conditions further compound this harm by failing to remedy social, political, and environmental injustices that contribute to harm. As Sandra's and Brisa's experiences show, policies of exclusion of immigrant populations contributed to economic insecurity and a lived sense of instability. Sandra experienced this precarity beginning in childhood, growing up undocumented. Brisa experienced more intense feelings of insecurity at the time of the research, although as a recent immigrant, these emotions did not characterize her earlier life. Yet, both women went on to develop preeclampsia. The insufficient safety nets during the pandemic further exacerbated experiences of stress, and Janeth's resulting emotions included contemplating suicide while pregnant and postpartum. The lack of postpartum employment protections exacerbated the harm that resulted from Lupe's postpartum preeclampsia. Postpartum preeclampsia may be especially dangerous for women with CHIP Perinatal who have limited coverage following the delivery, as they may be less likely to seek care for concerning symptoms. While preeclampsia may inevitably occur even among the most affluent members of society, the high burden of the condition among marginalized and racialized groups in the border region calls for attention to the social and environmental context and the policies that have produced this context. From this perspective, the toll of preeclampsia is the end result of a series of harmful policies.

4

Conjugated Harm and Pregnancy during the Pandemic

In March 2020, initial pandemic lockdowns led Diana and her boyfriend to both lose their jobs. Without stable income, they struggled to care for their three children, ages three, two, and one. Neither Diana nor her boyfriend were able to receive unemployment benefits. Her boyfriend had been working full time, but his company classified him as an independent contractor and therefore self-employed. Hypothetically, he could have qualified for unemployment. Although the details were unclear to Diana, he was not able to provide the documents he needed to file for unemployment. Diana had technically resigned from her part-time job, which she believed made her ineligible. Her resignation came after her children's daycare closed and she had no other childcare options. For Diana, leaving work was more than a lost income. Compounding her sense of loss was the fact that gaining employment and earning her own income had enabled her to leave a previously abusive relationship.

Diana likely could have qualified for unemployment. Prior to the pandemic, she would have only qualified for unemployment in Texas if she had resigned to care for a child with a medical illness. However, the Pandemic Unemployment Assistance (PUA) program did allow benefits for those unable to work because of school and childcare closures. The exclusion of both Diana and her boyfriend from unemployment may reflect systematic patterns of bureaucratic violence, similar to those discussed in chapter 1 related to continuous Medicaid coverage during the public health emergency. A *ProPublica* investigation (Beauvais and Ferman 2021) found that the Texas Workforce Commission (TWC) was systematically denying unemployment claims for any minor error, giving applicants little explanation as to what they needed to correct. Those with denied claims had to navigate a complicated bureaucracy that they often did not understand. Many, including Diana's boyfriend, may have believed they simply did not qualify. As Diana's experience suggests, many people were unaware of the expanded benefits that could have helped them in a time of crisis.

As the couple struggled to make ends meet, Diana's boyfriend tried desperately to find a new job, but he was without stable employment for four months. Given their precarious childcare situation, Diana was unable to seek steady employment. In the meantime, they both worked odd jobs, mostly cleaning houses and doing yardwork. Diana felt limited to taking jobs that allowed her to bring her children with her. When her boyfriend did find a steady job, it paid significantly less than his previous job. Their monthly household income had dropped from $2,600 prior to the pandemic to $1,600 in April 2021. A year after being out of the workforce, Diana lamented about the persistent economic hardship produced by her continued inability to work, saying, "I think that my boyfriend tries, because he works all day, but he's not making enough money. He gets frustrated and he doesn't tell me. Then I get frustrated 'cause I want to work, but I can't, 'cause how can anybody help me with the kids? I want to go to school. I want to do a lot of things to be better, like, to look for a better job. But I can't 'cause I don't have daycare."

Diana emphasized their economic struggles, especially during the earliest months of the pandemic, saying, "It was very frustrating. We could pay rent or buy food or pay the bills." But they could not pay for everything. They looked for help wherever they could get it, but this support was not enough to enable them to feel secure. Food pantries became a lifeline. In addition to relying on food pantries, Diana applied for food stamps. It took six months for Health and Human Services (HHS) to approve their application. According to Diana, HHS kept requesting additional documentation. Staffing shortages and overwhelming demand at HHS may have contributed to this situation. Diana and her boyfriend also sought utility assistance through a community organization, but by the time someone processed their materials, the organization had run out of funds. Diana should have been receiving child support from the father of her three-year-old. However, the father had a history of abusing Diana and continued to find ways to torment her, which included not paying child support. Given the abuse and his lack of involvement as a father, Diana had initially sought full custody of their child. Her ex, in an effort to maintain joint custody, threatened to call Immigration and Customs Enforcement on Diana's undocumented brother-in-law if she did not record a video of herself recanting her claims of domestic abuse. Because Diana gave into his threats, she was unsuccessful in her attempt to gain sole custody. The father rarely visited his daughter, and instead, exercised his custody by refusing to sign their daughter's passport application—a significant inconvenience for Diana given her extensive family network in Juárez.

In the midst of her household's economic struggles, Diana discovered she was pregnant in January 2021. Although she was concerned about the health of her baby, especially since she knew she had not been eating well, she delayed seeking prenatal care. The media images of overwhelmed hospitals made her feel panic at the thought of going to a doctor's office. As the vaccine became available and infection rates began to decline, Diana called several hospitals to schedule an appointment. The first two hospital systems she called told her that there were long waiting lists for all of their providers. University Medical Center (UMC), the county safety-net hospital, was the third hospital she called and the only one able to schedule her for an appointment. At her first prenatal visit, she was twenty-nine weeks pregnant and her provider informed her that she might have preeclampsia. It is likely that a high blood pressure reading at her first visit may have led her provider to tell her she needed additional monitoring for potential preeclampsia. Fortunately, according to Diana's medical records, she did not go on to develop preeclampsia.

Diana's experiences reflect some of the patterns of hardship for pregnant people during the pandemic, especially prior to the widespread availability of the vaccine. In El Paso, between March 1 and May 1, 2020, over 50,000 people filed unemployment claims out of a workforce of about 350,000 (Kladzyk 2020). This figure does not account for people who did not apply for unemployment based on the assumption they would not qualify for benefits. As our interviews showed, many people were unaware of pandemic provisions that expanded qualification criteria, leading them to think they would not have a successful case. Further, the application process in Texas was so burdensome and confusing that it created bureaucratic disenfranchisement and de facto exclusion from benefits for many people (see Beauvais and Ferman 2021).

Diana's exit from the workforce in response to limited childcare options was a part of what journalist Amanda Holpuch (2020) described as the "shecession," in which already fragile and insufficient safety nets collapsed and low-wage working mothers with young children disproportionately shouldered the resulting caretaker burdens (Zanhour and McDaniel Sumpter 2022). Notably, by October 2020, four times as many women had left the workforce as men. Layoffs were disproportionately high among women and people of color. Yet, many of the low-income women leaving the workforce were unable to access unemployment. Although Diana felt forced to leave her job, the fact that she voluntarily resigned led her to believe she did not qualify for benefits.

As jobs vanished, so did savings, income available for household bills and food, and a sense of security. Diana's family had already been living paycheck to paycheck and quickly spiraled into crisis mode. Food distribution centers became a lifeline for Diana's family and others experiencing job loss. Food insecurity was telling of the consequences of the economic fallout. In the United States, the prevalence of food insecurity went from 10.5 percent before the pandemic to 23 percent following initial lockdowns. Nearly one-third of households with children were food insecure (Dolin et al. 2021). Immigration concerns further exacerbated food insecurity by posing limits on access to Supplemental Nutrition Assistance Program (SNAP) benefits such as food stamps. Mixed-status families that operate as household units felt the reverberations of these policies, as heads of household with an insecure status often fear utilizing the benefits available to their US-citizen children (Castañeda 2019).

Years following initial pandemic layoffs, economic struggles persisted. As the economy reopened, initial job growth was higher in low-wage sectors that had experienced disproportionate job loss early in the pandemic (Fujita 2022). Further, as pandemic restrictions eased, inflation skyrocketed, giving households less purchasing power (Bohn and Lafortune 2022). It is telling that the main supplier to food banks and pantries throughout the city went from disbursing 32.5 million pounds of food in 2019 to nearly 140 million pounds in 2020 and 2021 respectively (El Pasoans Fighting Hunger 2023). Diana and her family were among those who regularly waited in line at area food banks, even as the economy rebounded.

Prior to the pandemic, El Paso had a higher rate of poverty than state and national rates combined with a high percentage of the population lacking health insurance. There was also a preexisting high burden of food insecurity, especially in the most marginalized sectors of the city (Núñez-Mchiri, Riviera, and Marrufo 2017). Even prior to the pandemic, these structural factors contributed to health vulnerabilities that may produce maternal and infant health risks. As El Paso became one of the hardest hit US cities during the fall 2020 wave of COVID-19, local health care infrastructures operated in crisis mode. The context of overwhelmed hospitals and fears of getting sick from going to prenatal appointments led to increased rates of inadequate prenatal care, further exacerbating structural risks (Goyal et al. 2021). During the fall of 2020, as El Paso entered its worst wave of the pandemic, the clinic where we recruited participants was often empty. Clinic staff began double and triple booking appointment slots to offset the number of patients who did not show up to their prenatal visits. Some women, like Diana, did not even schedule prenatal appointments until late in their pregnancies out of fear of entering medical facilities.

The various hardships Diana faced during the pandemic constitute what I call *conjugated harm*. In using the term conjugated harm, I bring attention to the manifestations of conjugated oppression (Bourgois 1988) and structural vulnerability (Quesada, Hart, and Bourgois 2011). Philippe Bourgois uses the term conjugated oppression to show how individual experiences of oppression may be fundamentally different based on various dimensions of their social position. Like other intersectional approaches, conjugated oppression considers how multiple factors related to a person's social status can generate interlocking sources of marginalization. Conjugated oppression also considers how social ideologies, such as those that naturalize exclusion based on a person's immigration status, are essential to how oppression persists.[1] This oppression produces structural vulnerabilities that put marginalized groups and individuals at increased risk of emotional, social, and physical harms.

I use the term *conjugated harm* to capture the ways systems of oppression contribute to harm in relation to a person's various social positions within a given context and period of time. Doing so emphasizes why the effects of the pandemic created disproportionate harm for some people based on preexisting structural vulnerabilities. For example, it was one thing to lose a job during the pandemic. Not being able to access unemployment benefits because of labor or immigration policies further entrenched the potential harm that followed a job loss.

In what follows, I turn my attention to the emotional experience of pregnancy during the pandemic, attending to the contextual and temporal dimensions of these emotions. Emotional suffering is a potent register of structural vulnerability as it reflects the subjective experience of resulting harms. Diana's emotions—frustration, panic, and fear, to name a few—reflect how the pandemic exacerbated her preexisting structural vulnerabilities in ways that caused her disproportionate harm. As such, I engage with some of the most salient emotions that women used to describe their emotional states while pregnant during the pandemic: anxiety, despair, frustration, and gratitude. While most of these emotions reflect states of distress, I include gratitude to show how various aspects of a person's position and social relationships had the potential to offer relief and foster resilience in conditions of hardship.

The terms I use to capture emotional states came partially through women's own words to describe their mental status and, to a lesser degree, partially through my own grouping of closely related nomenclatures that women used. There are also linguistic nuances to consider. For example, despair does not fully capture the sentiment expressed through the Spanish word *desesperación*. In English, women often expressed feelings of depression or hopelessness in similar ways to how women used *desesperación* in Spanish. In both Spanish and English, women often expressed feelings of frustration and a sense of being trapped in similar ways. Situating these emotional expressions in relation to contextual factors is revealing of how and why the pandemic generated a disproportionate burden of conjugated harm in the border region.

The Local Biology of Emotions and Conjugated Harm

In El Paso, preexisting struggles within the border context contributed to how people emotionally experienced the pandemic. The extended closure of the border disrupted familial ties, especially for those with family members lacking US citizenship or legal permanent residency. It is difficult to find estimates on the number of families who may identify as transnational, but the sheer number of people who crossed the border regularly prior to the closure is telling. Prepandemic, northbound cross-border traffic at El Paso ports of entry included twenty thousand pedestrians and thirty-five thousand cars per day (US DOT 2017).[2]

Immigration policies also have reverberations throughout the community. Out of a population of 867,947 in El Paso County, an estimated 52,000 US citizens live in a household with an undocumented person (Conner 2021). Beyond the household level, the effects of immigration policies are often diffuse and hard to pinpoint. Diana expressed no immigration-related concerns for her immediate family; it was her sister's husband who was undocumented. Yet, if her sister's husband were to be deported, it would have broken up her sister's family. The threat of this rupture was enough for Diana to give into her abuser's demands, further exacerbating her own vulnerabilities. Diana never even told her sister what had happened.

The healthcare infrastructure in El Paso also faced unique strains produced by regional patterns. Prepandemic, El Paso already had a chronic shortage of providers and significant portions of the county had the designation of Medically Underserved Areas (HRSA 2023). That health care institutions in El Paso serve populations in two countries exacerbates provider shortages. Although Mexican nationals could not easily cross during the border closure, there is a significant population of US residents and citizens residing in Mexican border cities. These individuals could continue to cross the border and, in the context of a health emergency, were at times inclined to use US emergency rooms over Mexican ones.

These contextual factors generated a particular set of structural circumstances that are unique to border communities. The long-term closure of the border disrupted family unity and cut people off from important sources of social support. Immigration issues exacerbated economic fallout, even for individuals with more diffuse social connections to precariously documented individuals. The overwhelmed hospital systems contributed to disruptions to prenatal care. The concept of local biologies is useful for understanding how these local dynamics shaped the emotional experience of the pandemic, as emotions are situational and in part a product of what is happening in a person's social world.

There are also temporal dimensions to consider, as the pressures produced by the pandemic evolved. Vaccine availability was a significant turning point as it mitigated some of the health threats of COVID-19. Although the vaccine became widely available in El Paso in late winter and spring of 2021, the vulnerabilities produced by the pandemic continued, especially for pregnant people. National data showed slow vaccine uptake among pregnant people (Bhattacharya et al. 2022), and we found a similar pattern among our participants. Even women who were otherwise enthusiastic about getting the COVID-19 vaccine often decided to wait until after the birth to get the vaccine. This decision came largely out of a fear that the vaccine could potentially harm the baby, despite mounting evidence that the risks posed by COVID-19 infection during pregnancy were far greater than potential risks from vaccination. The especially high rate of vaccine hesitancy among pregnant people of color is in part a consequence of a lack of trust in health care institutions that have a historical legacy of exploitation and abuse of communities of color (Nephew 2021). As many pregnant women delayed getting the vaccine, they described patterns of continued self-isolation to protect themselves and the baby. This at times included remaining out of the workforce despite economic hardships. Vaccination delays extended the emotional and economic toll of the pandemic for pregnant people, even as society entered a new normal.

Emotional Manifestations of Conjugated Harm

Temporal and contextual factors are important for understanding women's emotional experiences. Early in the pandemic, when there was confusion and a lack of data on the virus itself, panic and anxiety profoundly marked women's experiences. As the pandemic persisted, continued economic pressures, a lack of support with childcare, bearing witness to suffering, and continued fears of infection marked women's emotional states.

Anxiety

"This pandemic changed me completely. It made me hysterical and scared, especially because I studied nursing," Fabiola explained in November 2021, during the second trimester of pregnancy with her third child, which was also her second baby born during the pandemic. She had another baby in June 2020 and also had a seven-year-old.

Fabiola's life straddled both sides of the border. She was thirty-one years old when she became pregnant with her third child and had been a US resident for nearly two decades, since her father was able to gain residency and later sponsor his immediate family members. Since establishing US residency, Fabiola spent various spans of her childhood on different sides of the border. As an adult, she lived primarily in Juárez, but would periodically spend extended periods of time residing with her parents in El Paso in order to fulfill the conditions required to maintain her permanent residency status. Her time in El Paso strategically included the months leading up to the births of her children to ensure that she gave birth on US soil. Complicating matters, however, was the fact that her husband only had a border crossing card. During normal times, this was sufficient for allowing the couple to see each other frequently when Fabiola was staying in El Paso. The border closure, however, significantly ruptured their family unity leading up to the births of their younger children.

When Fabiola became pregnant with her second child in 2019, she began prenatal care in Juárez with plans to relocate to El Paso in the final month of pregnancy. She also planned for her husband to join her. In March 2020, when Fabiola was in the final trimester of the pregnancy, it became clear that crossing the border was going to become more complicated and she decided to go stay with her parents before the border closed. After relocating, she knew she could apply for CHIP Perinatal to continue her prenatal appointments, as she did with her previous pregnancy. However, she was terrified she would contract COVID-19 if she visited a doctor. Instead, she went her final stretch of pregnancy without a prenatal appointment and waited until she went into labor to go to the hospital. With her husband unable to cross the border, her mother served as her birth companion. Of the birth, she said, "I felt panicked to be in the hospital with so many people and everything with the virus."

As the pandemic continued, so did Fabiola's fears and anxiety. She went on to explain that as a nurse and mother, she could not get sick. She needed to be well enough to care for everyone else. Her entire family did in fact get sick with COVID-19 in November 2020. Her six-month-old and seven-year-old only had mild symptoms. Her husband had trouble breathing and low oxygen saturation, but he was not sick enough to go to the hospital, at least not at that moment during the pandemic when overloaded hospitals in Juárez could only admit the sickest patients. Fabiola described her symptoms as mild, yet her fears were intense. Her subsequent recovery from COVID-19 did little to alleviate her pandemic anxiety. Instead, she explained, "From there, I started having bouts of anxiety. For any symptom I had, I thought it was COVID again and that I would die. All of this caused me a lot of anxiety. Then, finally, all of that that [fear of the pandemic] went away, but the anxiety stayed." When I interviewed Fabiola over a year and a half into the pandemic, she explained that she was no longer as fearful as she was earlier in the pandemic, but her anxieties had shifted to having concerns about everything with her children.

The border context is significant for understanding the array of factors that contributed to Fabiola's persistent anxiety. For the final stages of her second pregnancy and most of her third pregnancy, the US-Mexico border split Fabiola's family. Although she returned to live with her husband in Juárez after the birth of their second child, when she became pregnant again, she quickly moved back to El Paso. Part of her decision to do this was to avoid border crossing challenges during the extended closure of the border. As a US permanent resident seeking essential health services, she maintained a legal right to cross. Yet, she lacked the full protections of citizenship and feared that a Border Patrol agent could simply deny her entry. Her decision to remain in El Paso came at a cost, however, as it meant an extended period of separation from her husband who would again miss the birth of their child.

Temporality is important for understanding the intensity of Fabiola's anxiety. When Fabiola's family fell ill with COVID-19 in November 2020, the hospitals in both Juárez and El Paso were overflowing. In El Paso, hospitals set up outdoor tents as waiting areas. The situation in Juárez, where the couple resided at the time, was perhaps more dire. The Mexican public health sector had established mobile hospitals, and the city cemeteries preemptively began digging graves to bury the unclaimed bodies. Fabiola's assertion that her husband was not "sick enough" to go to the hospital despite his escalating symptoms reflects the stories circulating on both sides of the border of people who were initially sent home, told they were not sick enough for admission, only to have to return in a more severe condition.

Patterns of cross-border health care utilization may have also contributed to Fabiola's fears. In early November 2020, an El Paso first responder alerted the *El Paso Times* to the number of emergency calls they were receiving to take severely ill people from US ports of entry to local hospitals. This account hinted at accusations that Juárez residents were exploiting US health services, given the more fragile and underresourced system in Mexico. Follow-up investigations revealed that nearly all of those transported by ambulance to local hospitals were US citizens or permanent residents. Fabiola and her children would have legal rights to engage in this same practice—if they were able to pay for the care. Her husband, however, would have been restricted to care in Juárez given his lack of US residency.

While Fabiola described her emotions though the label of anxiety, she never received a medical diagnosis for this condition. The same was true for many other women who described feeling anxiety, *nervios*, or otherwise anxious states. *Nervios* is an idiom of distress among people of Latin American origin that often overlaps with anxiety, depression, and panic (Guarnaccia 1993). The absence of a medical diagnosis does not imply a person's emotions are not real. Anxiety may be underdiagnosed in populations with limited access to health care (Stockdale et al. 2008). Beyond that, anxiety exists on a continuum, and not all manifestations of it are debilitating or severe enough to result in a diagnosis (Siddaway, Taylor, and Wood 2018).

Isabela, however, had a medical diagnosis of anxiety. She described how her anxiety emerged following the mass shooting on August 3, 2019, that left twenty-three people dead. That morning, her husband left home to buy groceries at the Cielo Vista Walmart—what would soon become the site of the racially driven massacre. Isabela stayed at home with their three-day-old baby and toddler. At some point, she picked up her phone and saw an emergency text alert reporting an active shooter in the Cielo Vista area. The details were vague. News outlets at first conveyed conflicting details over where the emergency calls were coming from, as some initial reports suggested the shooter was in the nearby mall. As Isabela waited for details, in a panic, she tried desperately to call her husband. Her calls and messages would not go through. The area cell phone towers could not support the number of calls people were making. Soon, the media confirmed mass casualties at the Walmart where Isabela's husband had gone to shop. Two hours later, she finally heard back from her husband. He had never made it to Walmart, and instead, had been trapped in the traffic produced by the chaos. Among those murdered were a young couple who had shielded their two-month-old baby from bullets. Isabela said, "After the shooting, I just became more aware that we're not entirely safe all the time. I just keep thinking of keeping my kids safe, keeping everyone safe."

It took months for Isabela to understand how her emotions were continuing to affect her following the shooting. After family members approached her with their concerns, she agreed to seek therapy. However, without health insurance, she had limited options. Her preferred method of treatment was counseling, but she had trouble getting an appointment for reduced-cost services. Instead, she was only able to get an appointment with a physician who prescribed her medication. Mentally, the medication helped her. Physically, it made her feel terrible, and "getting out of bed hurt." As a result, she stopped taking the prescription. By that time, the pandemic was in full swing, and Isabela continued to find it impossible to get an appointment for counseling. The combination of the shooting and fears over potential exposure to the virus made her home feel like the only safe space for her.

Given her anxiety, Isabela and her family remained isolated as much as possible during the first year of the pandemic. Yet, after exposure through extended family, everyone in her household contracted COVID-19 in November 2020. Fortunately, no one required hospitalization and the one-year-old was asymptomatic. Isabela, however, had lingering gastrointestinal (GI) symptoms that lasted into her subsequent pregnancy. When we first spoke at the beginning of her second trimester in April 2021, she was extremely worried that she had not gained any weight. Her lasting COVID-19 symptoms made it difficult for her to have an optimal pregnancy diet, explaining, "Eating is painful. Not eating is painful." The lack of nutrition contributed to her having anemia and left her exhausted, without energy. It also fueled her anxiety. Her midwife was able to get her an appointment with a GI specialist and counselor, with both covered under Medicaid for Pregnant Women. This additional care that she had been unable to access while uninsured prior to her pregnancy helped Isabela physically and emotionally throughout the remainder of her pregnancy. Isabela was more at ease in the second half of her pregnancy and her baby arrived full-term at a healthy weight. Postpartum, she felt like her anxiety was continuing to improve, especially since the vaccine was preventing severe infection. However, she was worried that she would lose access to her therapy services once her Medicaid expired. Like other women previously discussed, Isabela was under the impression that her Medicaid would expire soon after the birth of her child.

Both Isabela and Fabiola expressed anxiety over seeking health care services, especially during periods of time when COVID-19 patients overwhelmed local hospitals. While this context delayed Isabela's ability to find mental health care and services for her lingering COVID-19 symptoms, it did not delay her initiation of prenatal care. Given the timing of Fabiola's pregnancies, the pandemic altered her prenatal care for her first pregnancy, but not her second. Anxiety, and other emotions women described in relation to anxiety, fundamentally shaped how women navigated health care structures during pregnancy.

Despair

Borderlands scholars and journalists frequently refer to El Paso's Segundo Barrio neighborhood as "the other Ellis Island." Segundo Barrio residents, both today and historically, have overwhelmingly been recent immigrants from Mexico, with the first wave settling in the 1910s during the Mexican Revolution. In the 1930s, developers built tenements to house Mexican laborers. Most of these buildings lacked water and heat until community protests in the 1970s resulted in ordinances requiring landlords to update their properties. Many of these tenement buildings remain occupied today with a combination of longtime residents and new waves of immigrants. In recent years, the Segundo Barrio has been listed as one of the poorest, but also one of the friendliest, neighborhoods in the United States (Ovalle 2020).

The US-Mexico border fence marks the southern boundary of this poor and friendly neighborhood. The Donald Trump administration ordered an additional crowning of concertina wire to the top of the fence. Throughout the neighborhood, there is a constant presence of Border Patrol vehicles and helicopters overhead. Beginning in early 2023, military tanks and uniformed members of the National Guard formed an additional barrier between the Segundo Barrio and Mexico in response to the increase in migrants waiting to enter the United States.

Brisa lived in this militarized setting during most of her pregnancy. Her apartment was in sight of the border wall, and she described "feeling the presence of immigration [Border Patrol]" as causing *desesperación*, which included emotional and bodily reactions. These reactions were not only about her own fears of Border Patrol stopping her but also from witnessing the experiences of other migrants. She regularly watched people cross the border, knowing she could not offer help to them because of her own status. She explained her emotions that resulted: "One day after I saw people crossing, I had these strong feelings for two days. I had many feelings, a lot of guilt. I dreamt they were my siblings. I felt selfish. I felt bad."

For Brisa, being undocumented was challenging, but she did not have intense feelings about her immigration status until the pandemic. She explained, "In the beginning [after migrating], I was more or less stable. But now, with the pandemic, I lost control. The pandemic changed everything. My life project of being self-sufficient. But it isn't just the pandemic. It's my economic situation, my legal status. My pregnancy has been beautiful, but it has been difficult." The combination of her immigration status and preexisting economic concerns compounded the negative ramifications of the pandemic for Brisa.

Brisa stated that the pandemic was not the best time to be pregnant. However, when she found out she was pregnant in the summer of 2020, the idea of having a baby brought new meaning to her life. This first pregnancy ended in a miscarriage, which she experienced as traumatic. When she quickly became pregnant a second time, she knew she would do whatever was necessary to protect the baby. Her desire to protect her child further exacerbated other vulnerabilities. After losing her jobs cleaning houses during lockdowns, she knew she needed other employment, but feared the consequences of working the jobs most readily available to her. In previous jobs, she regularly worked long hours, lifted heavy objects, and used strong chemicals—all activities she feared could contribute to another miscarriage. She also feared contracting COVID-19 while pregnant. A close friend had COVID-19 while pregnant and the birth occurred prematurely. Both Brisa and her friend attributed the premature birth to the COVID-19 infection. The hesitation over taking any job available to her resulted in continued economic deprivation. These financial struggles were a primary source of despair for Brisa throughout her pregnancy.

For Brisa, her sense of despair was bound up in her social position and the material realities of her life. She also linked despair to other emotions—guilt, fear, and depression. Notably absent were feelings of anger, which some women described as related to their despair. Anessa, for example, described despair resulting from not being able to work, financial strain, and having to live with her in-laws. Anessa's despair at times manifested as frustration and anger, as her situation led her to lose her temper over things that would not normally bother her. She moved into her in-laws' home, despite their lack of space, out of financial necessity. The pandemic lockdowns made this space feel even smaller, as there was no way to escape. For Anessa and others, despair and feeling trapped were overlapping emotions.

Feeling Trapped

"The pandemic made me feel trapped," explained Helena. In March 2020, Helena and her boyfriend Gustavo both lost their jobs. Helena had just found out she was pregnant with their first child. Neither Helena nor Gustavo was receiving unemployment. Helena decided to delay seeking work, concerned about the additional risks she would face if she were to get sick with COVID-19 while pregnant. Gustavo, who was undocumented, tried desperately to find a job. For over a year, he was only able to piece together temporary jobs. During that time, the couple made ends meet on roughly $800 a month. To survive on this income, they moved in with Gustavo's parents. Gustavo's sister and her children were already living in the same household. The two school-age children were home all day for virtual schooling. Helena described the living situation as "like being in a prison. A disaster." Her only escape was to visit her own family. Although she was grateful to have the support of Gustavo's family, her situation led her to feel trapped in multiple ways, including suffering economic constraints, sharing the same household with extended family, and feeling like it was impossible to get a new job while pregnant.

Multigenerational households are common in El Paso. There are economic advantages to such household structures. Living with extended family members offers a way to pool resources and manage economic hardships in a region with a high rate of poverty. Many women we interviewed moved in and out of households with extended family members, including in-laws. Some of this was in response to economic pressures produced by the pandemic. The overall circumstances of women's lives contributed to how they felt about such living arrangements.

While Helena had a precarious economic situation leading her to move in with Gustavo's family, she did have some degree of privilege conferred by her residency status. After her father had the opportunity to adjust his status, he sponsored Helena's residency application. She had been living in the United States for just under five years at the time of our interview. While she felt frustrated by her job loss, she did not have the added struggle of lacking work authorization, although Gustavo lacked these legal protections. Women without permanent residency or citizenship often faced additional constraints that exacerbated their sense of entrapment at home.

In early 2021, Anessa relocated from Juárez to El Paso. She had just married Alonzo, a US citizen who lived in El Paso, whom she had met through her church. In Juárez, she had recently completed her university degree in engineering. She had always worked while she pursued her higher education, although she had not yet found a job in her profession while still in Juárez. Anessa and Alonzo decided to move in with Alonzo's parents in El Paso following their marriage. Alonzo had never moved out of their house, and the couple hoped to save money to move into their own place. They also had legal fees to consider. Anessa was shocked when she initially looked into how much it cost to go through a lawyer to submit her application for permanent residency via marriage to a US citizen.

Shortly after settling into her in-laws' home, Anessa became pregnant. She was happy about the pregnancy, but despite her happiness at the prospect of motherhood, she quickly fell into a state of depression. She had wanted her mother and sister to be with her for the pregnancy, but she had no idea when she would see them again. The US-Mexico border remained closed, and only US citizens and permanent residents could cross easily. Anessa could not cross while waiting to adjust her immigration status. Her mother and sister could not cross, given they only had border crossing cards.

Anessa described her depression in relation to other emotions—anger, frustration, and a sense of despair. She ultimately pinpointed feeling trapped as the cause of these related emotions. At the time of our first interview in late summer of 2021, the situation with the pandemic was improving. Anessa had received the COVID-19 vaccine and new variants that could evade the vaccine had not yet become the dominant strains. Her sense of feeling trapped was less about a need to continue isolating and more about not being able to work until after establishing legal residency and being cut off from her social network because of the extended border closure. She explained, "I was never home not doing anything [before the move to El Paso]. I was always studying or working. I was always able to be independent. Now, I am in the house all day. I feel very frustrated." While she described her in-laws as welcoming her and treating her well, she still felt like it was not her home and she longed for her own space and privacy. She did not share these feelings with her husband, worried he would think she regretted marrying him.

Gratitude

In the summer of 2020, Yolanda had finally secured stable work after years of part-time work as a substitute paraprofessional staff at her oldest child's school. Earlier that year, both her and her husband were completely out of work for over a month and worried about supporting their eight- and four-year-old children. With virtual schooling, there was little need for substitutes and Yolanda lost her income. Yolanda's husband worked in the food service industry, which experienced some of the most widespread layoffs early in the pandemic. Yolanda believed she did not qualify for unemployment because of her temporary employee status, although she may have in fact qualified. Her husband delayed applying, optimistic that he would not be out of work for long. He was indeed one of the first employees his restaurant called back, and they tasked him with managing curbside service. During the employment lapse, Yolanda's family struggled, but they were able to pool resources with her in-laws who lived next door to make sure that everyone had what they needed. "Thankfully, we managed through," she said.

Given the dramatic increase in food insecurity at the national level, federal funding supported curbside breakfast and lunch distribution for children through local schools throughout the summers of 2020 and 2021 and while schools remained virtual for most of the 2020–21 school year. The school where Yolanda had worked as a substitute was hiring part-time food service workers starting in the summer of 2020, with the likelihood that the job would transition to full time during the upcoming school year. Yolanda was ecstatic when she received a job offer. Complicating matters, however, was that she discovered she was pregnant just weeks into her new job. Her boss told her that she could take time off without losing her job, although the time would be unpaid, given she had not been a full-time employee long enough to accrue much sick leave. While Yolanda expressed concerns over the need to return to work quickly following the birth, she also felt like the situation would be manageable, even if not ideal. Her mother-in-law lived next door and was happy to take care of the baby so that Yolanda could return to work.

While Yolanda had experienced hardships throughout the pandemic, she was grateful for the social support network that she had. She also referenced many people who had it much harder than she did. If the pandemic had occurred earlier in Yolanda's life, she knew she would have faced much more challenging circumstances because of her past immigration status. Although Yolanda had lived in El Paso since she was eleven years old, she had arrived with her mother without documentation. It was not until 2018 that Yolanda was able to adjust her immigration status via marriage to a US citizen. She was grateful that her residency status gave her a greater feeling of security than she had with her previous pregnancies. During her first pregnancy, she was unaware that she could apply for CHIP Perinatal until late in her pregnancy and significantly delayed seeking prenatal care. For her most recent pregnancy, she felt well cared for, even though she continued to have limited coverage under CHIP Perinatal since she had not yet met the length of residency requirements to qualify for Medicaid.

Yolanda, like many women, faced challenges during the pandemic. Yet, knowing how much other people were struggling and having the sense that her situation could be much worse armed her with a sense of gratitude that helped her navigate these challenges. Talia echoed this sentiment saying, "I know a lot of people lost their jobs, and I know there were lots of struggles. I mean, thank God for me, nothing bad happened." While Talia stated that "nothing bad happened," she did lose two different jobs because of the circumstances of getting pregnant during the pandemic. When she found out she was pregnant in early 2021, she was working twelve-hour shifts at a fast-food restaurant. The long shifts were in part a consequence of the labor shortage in low-paying jobs as the economy was reopening. She knew that being on her feet for so long every day, combined with occupational risks of COVID-19 exposure, would not be good for the pregnancy. Hiding her pregnancy in order to find a new job, a food warehouse hired her. While she was still in her probationary period, she fell ill with COVID-like symptoms, but tested negative for COVID-19. She struggled to recover given that she was also dealing with morning sickness. Due to the missed work, her employer quickly terminated her.

After losing the second job, Talia's parents and boyfriend intervened. They urged her to take a break from working to enjoy the pregnancy, promising to support her financially. Talia's boyfriend was a soldier stationed at Fort Bliss in El Paso. He received deployment orders shortly after Talia became pregnant but promised financial support, giving Talia his credit card to buy whatever she needed for herself and the baby. She then moved back to her parents' house so that she would not have to stay alone at her boyfriend's house while he was away for most of her pregnancy. She described feeling simultaneously suffocated and supported by her family's efforts to ensure she had a healthy pregnancy. Talia laughed as she said, "My mom like suddenly became a doctor when I got pregnant." Ultimately, although Talia may have been vulnerable to the challenges created by becoming pregnant during the pandemic, the relatively privileged statuses of those around her helped ensure her well-being.

Talia and Yolanda both faced circumstances during their pregnancies that could have led to catastrophic situations in their lives. Lost jobs and unplanned pregnancies put them both in vulnerable positions. Their support systems enabled them to navigate difficult circumstances, ensuring their economic and emotional stability. Their familial ties in particular protected them from more profound experiences of conjugated harm. Emotionally, this generated feelings of gratitude in place of what could have otherwise been emotional distress.

Conjugated Harm and Reproductive Violence

Job loss, economic instability, food insecurity, feelings of loss and isolation, and more limited access to health care because of overstrained resources characterized the early stages of the COVID-19 pandemic.

While these concerns plagued the entire United States, certain issues were more acute in the border context. The extended border closure, amplification of immigration-related concerns, and preexisting structural vulnerabilities led the pandemic to have a particularly high toll in El Paso, not just in terms of the death count, but also in terms of the social and emotional suffering that ensued.

Analytically, conjugated harm offers a framework for connecting compounding structural vulnerabilities to reproductive violence. A person's gender, race, social class, and immigration status are among the oppressive domains exacerbated by experiences of economic crisis, hunger, and limited access to care. Emotions are an indicator of women's subjective experiences of this harm. Beyond that, as we saw earlier, there are also deeper health consequences related to emotional responses. Further, the emotional, physical, and social dimensions of injury limit a person's ability to experience pregnancy and raise a child in dignified conditions of their choosing. In what follows, I move into a discussion of clinical encounters and postpartum experiences. Clinical encounters, even when positive, only have limited potential for ameliorating the harms generated by broader structures of oppression. Postpartum experiences reveal the lasting effects of the crises that families fell into during earlier phases of the pandemic.

5

Finding Compassionate Care

In June of 2020, Brisa suspected she was pregnant for the first time. Although she had not planned the pregnancy, she was happy. At thirty-six years old, she had long wanted a child but had never had a serious relationship in her rural village in Mexico. After immigrating to the United States, she began seeing a man whom she had met through friends. One morning several weeks after her first missed period, she began experiencing intense cramping and bleeding. Having never sought medical care in the United States before, she was unsure of where she could go. Her shared apartment was near a group of hospitals and medical complexes, so that evening, she set out in that direction. El Paso was in the midst of an intense heat wave and the temperature had spiked to 105 degrees by late afternoon. The temperature was just beginning to drop. Brisa first looked for a smaller doctor's office, but they all appeared closed. She then entered what was likely an urgent care facility based on the details she recounted. There, a receptionist told her they could not see her because she did not have insurance. They instead directed her to the emergency room of a nearby private hospital. In the emergency room, she informed the receptionist that she did not have insurance, but they accepted her, along with the $300 she had brought with her.

Despite paying a large sum of money, Brisa felt neglected by the medical personnel who attended her. A technician came in to perform an ultrasound. When Brisa frantically asked how the baby was, the technician told her she had to speak to the doctor whom she had seen upon admission. The doctor never returned. Instead, a nurse told her not to worry and that she could return if she bled through more than three sanitary napkins that night. This nurse then discharged her. When Brisa left the emergency room, she still did not know the status of her baby.[1] The next morning, her body released larger fibrous blood clots. When she called her mother sobbing, it was her mother who confirmed what Brisa had feared. She was having a miscarriage.

Brisa said, "I didn't want to accept it. I felt like my soul had left me." Feeling like she still needed confirmation, she thought about going to a hospital again, but said, "I didn't want anything to do with hospitals because I did not feel I had help or care." At the urging of a friend, however, Brisa went to University Medical Center (UMC), the county safety-net hospital. In the medical encounter that followed, Brisa described a completely different experience than what had transpired in her previous emergency room visit: "The treatment was very different. Very humane and quick. All the doctors and nurses asked me how I was. I was worried about the bills, and they told me not to worry, that I could do a payment plan and they gave me information on how to get a discount." For follow-up care, she received a referral to a community clinic. At that clinic, she was happy to see the same midwife who had cared for her at UMC. The community clinic also provided her with a counseling session and encouraged her to return if she continued showing signs of depression. Just weeks later, she was pregnant again and immediately began prenatal care with the community clinic. The clinic staff helped her apply for CHIP Perinatal, and once approved, she began her prenatal appointments with the midwifery practice associated with UMC. Texas Tech University Health Science Center–El Paso, or simply Texas Tech, provides clinical services associated with UMC. Although locals often use "UMC" and "Texas Tech" interchangeably, technically, UMC is the county hospital system and Texas Tech encompasses the network of faculty and providers through the medical school. Brisa's first prenatal appointment was with the same Texas Tech midwife she had in her previous encounters at UMC and the community clinic.

Over multiple interviews, Brisa spoke of how she felt well cared for during her prenatal appointments and the birth. Despite numerous complications during the final stages of pregnancy and the birth, which included gestational diabetes, severe preeclampsia, a retained placenta that required manual removal, and postpartum hemorrhage, she described the birth as a "harmonious experience." When she began feeling nervous at the beginning of labor induction following her preeclampsia diagnosis, the nurse led her through breathing techniques that helped to calm her. She joyfully recounted that in the final stages of labor she was able to touch the baby's hair and see the head in a mirror between pushes. Feeling like care was accessible to her at UMC also made it easier for her to return when she had symptoms of postpartum preeclampsia. With dangerously high blood pressure, she remained hospitalized for another three days for monitoring and treatment. CHIP Perinatal did not cover her postpartum hospitalization; instead, Emergency Medicaid covered the costs. Her earlier encounters at UMC likely put her financial concerns at ease. Had Brisa felt unable to return due to economic concerns, the postpartum preeclampsia could have become more serious. Given her limited postpartum coverage, Brisa's midwife referred her back to the community clinic for counseling when she screened positive for postpartum depression at her postpartum visit. Brisa later returned to the community clinic for the COVID-19 vaccine.

Brisa's experiences show how a given health care institution and its employees can contribute to vastly different experiences of care for the same individual. It may come as a surprise that Brisa spoke so highly of her care as an uninsured patient at a public hospital, which was a stark contrast to the negligence she described when seeking care for a miscarriage at a private facility. Also striking is how little the pandemic seemed to alter the prenatal and birth care that Brisa received, given the potential for the pandemic to disrupt care in ways that could exacerbate obstetric violence (Sadler, Leiva, and Olza 2020). Certain institutional factors, especially the fact that Brisa had a midwife and encountered health care personnel who she felt empathized with her situation, played important roles in her overall experience.

Using the experiences of Brisa and four other women, I interrogate the role of providers and institutional factors in shaping women's experiences of obstetric care during the pandemic. These forces coalesced with women's various structural vulnerabilities and were fundamental to how they experienced obstetric care. To show the variability of individual experiences, and how contextual dimensions factored into their experiences, I include women with different positionalities. Before delving into their narratives, I discuss the history of efforts in providing reproductive health care to marginalized populations in El Paso and how this history has shaped current contexts of care. I also use interviews with providers to explain how policies in labor and delivery evolved as the pandemic unfolded in order to set the stage for analyzing individual experiences. Within my discussion of providers and institutional forces, I focus on midwives. Historically, midwifery has played a significant role in providing access to reproductive health services within an exclusionary health care system in the border region.

Midwifery in the Historical Context of Reproductive Care in El Paso

Central to Brisa's positive experiences of care was her use of midwives. The midwifery model of care attends to the holistic social, mental, and physical well-being during reproductive events, with a focus on empowerment, respect, and autonomy, alongside training to identify risks and intervene if necessary (Rooks 1999). This is a stark contrast to an overmedicalized model of birth that pathologizes normal physiological processes, which has historically characterized OB-GYN (doctor of obstetrics and gynecology) training and practice (Davis-Floyd 1992). While interventions such as C-sections, inducing labor, and augmenting labor are at times necessary and life-saving procedures, their widespread overuse in the United States and elsewhere is often more about giving control to physicians than prioritizing medical need. A consequence of this overmedicalization is increased potential for iatrogenic harm and traumatic birth experiences (Liese et al. 2021). Given the pushback against this overmedicalization, there have been some recent shifts as a part of OB-GYN training aimed at reducing interventions and providing more compassionate care. This has occurred alongside a shift in medicine that has responded to calls for cultural and structural competency as a part of medical training (Kleinman and Benson 2006; Metzl and Roberts 2014). However, there are still clearly patterned differences between midwifery and OB-GYN training and practice.

The distinct paradigms of midwifery and OB-GYN practice contribute to differential birth outcomes. Notably, births attended by midwives are less likely to involve unnecessary interventions and more likely to result in better birth outcomes for low and moderate risk pregnancies (MacDorman and Singh 1998). Despite different approaches to labor and birth, midwives and OB-GYNs often practice alongside each other, especially if a midwifery patient develops complications that require transfer to an OB-GYN. Further, within many medical schools, OB-GYN residents train under both midwives and physicians. Given the overlapping practice, there is evidence that having midwives present within a given hospital can lower the rate of C-sections, inductions, and labor augmentations, even among OB-GYN-attended births. This association suggests that having midwives present can contribute to institutional changes (Neal et al. 2019). Because of these patterns, many birth advocates support increased access to midwives as a way to promote humane approaches to childbirth.

Despite the more positive birth experiences associated with using a midwife, in 2018, midwives attended only 9 percent of births in the United States (Grünebaum et al. 2020). This is in large part a consequence of the reverberations of a history of smear campaigns that led to the marginalization of midwifery in the United States. Prior to the early twentieth century, midwives who learned their skills through apprenticeship and ancestral knowledge attended a majority of births in the United States. With the professionalization of medicine in the late nineteenth century, physicians began to view midwives and other traditional healers as a threat and engaged in strategies to delegitimize midwifery (Bonaparte 2015). Yet, women often resisted physician-led efforts that promoted having white male physicians attend births. In the Antebellum South, for example, white women continued to show a preference for using enslaved Black midwives for birth assistance. With the 1888 formation of the American Association of Obstetrics and Gynecology came more coordinated racially driven smear campaigns against the Black, Indigenous, and immigrant midwives who historically dominated the profession (Suarez 2020). There was significant regional variation in the effects of these campaigns. In some states, the American Medical Association (AMA) successfully lobbied for state legislation to ban midwifery and out-of-hospital births, yet midwifery endured, especially in rural areas and among poor people and people of color who either lacked trust in or had little access to physician services (Yoder and Hardy 2018).

Efforts to delegitimize midwives contributed to multiple trajectories within midwifery practice. For one, there were moves to formalize midwifery practice within biomedical contexts. This included establishing educational and credentialing systems for midwives within medical institutions. This approach catered to white nurses and actively excluded midwives of color. However, midwives who faced exclusion from formalized training continued to find ways to practice their profession (Dawley 2003). Midwives excluded from the biomedical realm also embarked upon professionalization efforts to maintain legitimacy through the establishment of formal apprenticeship programs.

Today, there are two types of midwives who commonly practice in the United States.[2] Certified Nurse Midwives (CNMs) train in nursing programs in a medical setting. This licensure allows them to attend low-risk births in a hospital setting and, in some states, in out-of-hospital contexts such as a birth center or at home. Certified Professional Midwives (CPMs) train and work outside of a hospital setting. CPMs can legally attend low-risk out-of-hospital births in Texas and thirty-five other states. Both CNMs and CPMs have an important presence in El Paso today, in part because of the historical significance of midwifery practice in the region.

The professionalization of medicine throughout the early twentieth century led hospitals to become the primary site of births, but only for some groups of women. In El Paso, racism toward Mexicans and Mexican Americans meant public health officials only encouraged white women to give birth in a hospital. In the US South, Jim Crow laws established segregated hospital systems for Black and white people. However, the same legal mechanisms for segregating racialized Mexican patients did not exist in Texas. Part of this is a reflection of the social construction of race. The US census designation of Mexicans as white did not match local ideologies that racialized Mexicans and Mexican Americans.

Borderlands historian Heather Sinclair (2016) shows how racist ideologies shaped the contexts of births during the early twentieth century. Given that national statistics did not distinguish between Mexican and Anglo patients, local physicians were concerned that the poorer birth outcomes among Mexicans would skew the statistics of white hospitals. As such, physicians and public health officials engaged in informal practices to keep Mexicans from birthing in hospitals. For one, hospitals would deny entry of "normal" cases of birth among Mexicans, as eugenics-inspired medicine defined the Mexican body as more "primitive" and fit for a home birth. When a hospital birth was necessary, doctors often kept Mexican patients out of maternity wards with Anglos and instead put them in wards with patients who were actively sick with contagious diseases that put mothers and their newborns at risk of infection. Over the next several decades, additional factors further deterred use of hospitals for birth among Mexican-origin women. Significantly, beginning in 1928 and throughout the Great Depression, the county hospital began reporting Mexican patients in the maternity wards to immigration officials (Sinclair 2016). Resulting deportations, which included US citizens, were part of wider anti-immigrant campaigns of this era (Balderrama and Rodríguez 2006).

Given the history of threats associated with using formal health services combined with outright denial of hospital care to Mexican patients, midwifery thrived. Yet, the racialized context of midwifery continued to influence the perceived legitimacy of midwives. Despite providing important medical services, public health officials blamed midwives for the high infant mortality rate in the region. In the 1920s, the infant mortality rate served as a pretext for limiting midwifery practice, despite no evidence of higher rates of stillbirths or infant deaths among midwifery attended births. Yet, these same public health officials simultaneously recognized the necessity of midwives within the community. To resolve this tension, public health officials established a local credentialing system that forced midwives to take a licensure test. However, this test was unavailable in Spanish, subsequently denying credentials to midwives with limited English proficiency. However, women continued to seek care from midwives who lacked formal credentials (Scragg 1981).

Alongside formal licensing of out-of-hospital midwives at the local level, efforts to integrate licensed nurse midwives into health care facilities increased. Beginning in 1937, the Houchen Settlement House, which served a primarily working-class Mexican immigrant neighborhood, added a maternity hospital that employed women to train and work as nurses and nurse midwives (Carr 2003). This maternity hospital had better birth outcomes than the county hospital that served primarily Anglo patients. Yet, rather than attributing these positive outcomes to the context of care women received from nurse midwives, leaders of the settlement house framed them in terms of eugenic ideas that imagined the Mexican body as more fit for the task of birth (Sinclair 2016).

While many states began banning midwifery in the mid-twentieth century, a 1956 court decision in Texas decided that midwifery did not fall into the practice of medicine, given that childbirth was a normal function (Scragg 1981). A series of subsequent state laws further enforced the distinction between midwives who had biomedical training in nursing and those who did not have this training. In response, there were efforts to professionalize apprenticeship-based training through the development of CPM programs.

As a part of this professionalization, important birth centers emerged in El Paso. These birth centers offered teaching and apprenticeship programs, leading the city to become one of the most important places nationally for the training of CPMs (Sinclair 2016).[3] As these birth centers thrived, the county hospital began integrating CNMs into the OB-GYN practice (Anchondo-Rivera 2016). Today, El Paso continues to have in-hospital- and out-of-hospital-based midwives. One unfortunate consequence of the historical context of midwifery in El Paso is there is still a lingering perception that midwives are for poor people, making it a substandard option, despite evidence of better birth outcomes among midwife-attended births.

Maternal Health Care in El Paso

At the beginning of my 2020–22 project, the Texas Tech midwifery practice associated with UMC had seven CNMs. Although there have been institutional efforts to expand midwifery services, the number of midwives began to decline throughout the pandemic. In addition to the challenges health care workers faced during the pandemic, there have been other barriers to recruiting and retaining midwives, especially given there is not a local CNM training program in El Paso.

Beyond UMC, the only other hospital in El Paso that has integrated midwives is William Beaumont Army Medical Center. As a military hospital, only those with military affiliation have access to their services. This makes UMC the only local hospital available to the wider population that has midwifery services. It is likely not a coincidence that UMC also has by far the lowest C-section rate of hospitals in El Paso. In 2019, 9.9 percent of births at UMC were delivered by C-section compared to rates of 26.2 percent and 22.3 percent at nearby private hospitals with large maternity wards (Martinez, McDonald, and Riker 2020). UMC has maintained this lower C-section rate despite being a Level IV maternal care facility, meaning they are equipped to care for the most complex births and are more likely to receive emergency transfers from other facilities and nearby rural areas.

Despite the local historical significance of midwifery, UMC has never had enough midwives to guarantee a patient that the birth will be attended by a midwife. Instead, a person could go their entire pregnancy receiving prenatal care from a midwife but have a resident or other physician attend the birth. While the residents receive part of their training under midwives, this scenario is not ideal for a person who has actively decided they prefer a midwife.

Among our research participants, approximately half of women used a midwife for their prenatal care. While some of these individuals had specifically requested a midwife, more often, they were simply taking the provider with whom they had been scheduled. When patients schedule their first visit, if they do not request a specific provider, they typically receive an appointment with the first available CNM or OB-GYN. CHIP Perinatal and Medicaid patients are often directed toward midwifery care. Although OB-GYNs within the practice will also take CHIP and Medicaid patients, they primarily see patients with private insurance. This institutional pattern is in part because publicly funded programs reimburse less than private insurance and midwifery care tends to be more cost effective (Baker et al. 2021). However, whether a patient receives an appointment with a midwife is at times contingent on provider availability and on who is scheduling appointments.

Beyond the hospital context, midwives have been integral to expanding reproductive health services through community clinics. Several Federally Qualified Health Centers (FQHCs) have secured grant funds to contract midwives from Texas Tech to provide regular reproductive health services, including prenatal care.[4] This is especially important for the provision of services not covered under the scope of CHIP Perinatal or Medicaid. For Brisa, after seeing a midwife at UMC following her miscarriage, she received a referral to a community clinic where she encountered the same midwife. This clinic assisted in her application for CHIP Perinatal when she became pregnant a second time, enabling her to have a smooth transition back to UMC/Texas Tech. When Brisa's CHIP Perinatal expired following the birth, she was able to return to this same clinic for follow-up care with her midwife.

This continuity of care was less likely for patients who used an OB-GYN. While some OB-GYNs do discuss community clinic options with their patients, many do not. When a person's coverage expires postpartum, they may be unaware of the services available at a community clinic. Without the advice from a midwife working in both settings and facilitating these connections, a person may be less likely to connect to follow-up services in a community clinic.

My aim in this discussion of midwifery is not to detract attention from the role of OB-GYNs and other health personnel. Rather, I wish to highlight that midwives have had a significant influence on the clinical contexts utilized by the women we interviewed. When I began listening to women's birth stories, I was expecting to hear more accounts of trauma and obstetric violence than what came through given patterns documented in hospital births in the United States, the compounding vulnerabilities generated by the pandemic, and the already marginalized positionalities of participants. While there were accounts of trauma and feelings of disempowerment, they were not as pervasive as I anticipated and many women described their birth experiences in positive ways. I am convinced that the influence of midwives within UMC was a significant factor in mitigating the potential for obstetric violence. The harms that women described were more often related to the contexts of their lives, with policies exacerbating the potential for these harms to manifest as poor health outcomes.

As Brisa's narrative shows, it is not just doctors and midwives that shape a person's overall experience of care. Other health personnel such as social workers, nurses, and billing and appointment coordinators all influence how people experience and utilize health services. Safety-net hospitals such as UMC may be more likely to be understaffed and underresourced, which creates challenges for providing quality care (Chatterjee et al. 2021). Further, patients seeking care through safety-net systems are more likely to be experiencing multiple structural vulnerabilities and limitations for accessing care. However, public hospitals that disproportionately serve marginalized populations may be more likely to adopt policies and promote practices that reflect structural and cultural competency in comparison to private for-profit institutions (Weech-Maldonado et al. 2012).[5]

For Brisa, considerations for her concerns over her ability to pay for services and offering information on applying to discount programs were important components of providing structurally competent care. Yet, different individuals within multiple layers of healthcare bureaucracy factor into if and how patients receive such information. For example, public safety-net hospitals typically offer charity care or discount programs. At UMC, patients residing in Mexico do not have access to the discount program that is available only to residents of El Paso County (who can qualify regardless of immigration status). Billing coordinators may exercise discretion in even informing patients of this program and may not offer information to patients that they assume reside in Mexico, instead telling them they must pay for services up front. Hospital employees may make incorrect assumptions about a person's ability to produce evidence of Texas residency. For example, in 2018, Celeste was undocumented, although she still had an unexpired border crossing card that she had used to enter the United States. She had declined coverage under CHIP Perinatal out of fear that using the program would make her a likely public charge and complicate her ability to adjust her immigration status in the future. Before leaving the hospital, a financial representative told her that she must pay her bill in full. Further, this representative told her that if she did not pay, Border Patrol would be able to see that she owed the hospital money and could revoke her visa. I have found little evidence to substantiate the financial representative's claims,[6] yet Celeste did not want to take any risks. She borrowed thousands of dollars from a family member to cover the cost of her C-section. The dramatically different experiences reported by Celeste and Brisa at the same institution reflect the degree of variation in how people may experience the same institutions as a consequence of the individuals with whom they interact.

Shifting Protocols during the Pandemic

Early in the pandemic, birth advocates expressed significant concern that the conditions of the pandemic would exacerbate the potential for obstetric violence. Especially during the first several months of the pandemic, hospital policies were constantly changing in ways that generated uncertainty for birthing people. In March 2020, when New York City became the epicenter of the pandemic in the United States, some hospitals began forcing birthing people to deliver alone. It was a measure aimed at reducing the risk of COVID-19 transmission, but which could easily contribute to an isolating or otherwise traumatic birth experience. Given the backlash from providers and patients, many hospitals quickly reversed course and amended policies to allow for one support person during the birth. However, policies related to the birthing person's COVID-19 status and NICU (neonatal intensive care unit) visitation continued to constantly change in relation to the conditions of the pandemic at a given location and time. Additionally, resource strains had the potential to produce neglect, as providers found themselves working in violent conditions. Narratives of health care worker heroism created challenges for questioning providers' decisions and demanding better care in the context of birth (Rice 2023).

Like hospital protocol everywhere, policies in labor and delivery wards in El Paso were constantly changing. Given that the first wave of COVID-19, in spring 2020, was relatively mild in El Paso, UMC never resorted to the outright denial of a birthing companion, unless the birthing person was COVID-19 positive upon admission. In the earliest months of the pandemic, UMC did not allow a COVID-19-positive mother to have a birthing companion, and immediately after the birth, separated the mother and baby. By the summer of 2020, a COVID-19-positive mother could have a support person. Babies were no longer separated from the mother, but instead placed in an Isolette in the same room, with no skin-to-skin contact permitted. During the subsequent fall surge, a COVID-19-positive mother once again had to deliver without a support person. A CNM who delivered babies under such circumstances described it as one of the most heartbreaking things she has had to do. These policies invariably created undue trauma, but also reflected initial uncertainties about mechanisms of transmission and levels of risk, especially for newborns (Shah and Didrik Saugstad 2021).

By early 2021, a COVID-19-positive mother could keep the baby in the room and have a support person as long as this person was not leaving and reentering. As we were finishing interviews in the summer of 2022, hospitals were beginning to allow two support people, in addition to support from a doula if the birthing person had hired one. Local hospitals had also stopped routine COVID-19 testing upon admission to labor and delivery unless the birthing person was symptomatic.

Even as policies relaxed, certain populations experienced greater potential for emotional trauma because of the COVID-19 policies that were in place. A CNM who often cared for pregnant inmates and immigration detainees commented on troubling patterns that were beyond the scope of what hospital policies could ameliorate. There was a period when prisons quarantined inmates following medical visits. The rationale for doing so was to avoid widespread outbreaks given the higher risk of COVID-19 transmission within prisons. However, medical isolation may mirror solitary confinement, which may lead to irreversible psychological harm (Cloud et al. 2020). To avoid periods of isolation, pregnant inmates began refusing prenatal care. Further, although the federal government has issued policies to direct the release of pregnant immigration detainees, Immigration and Customs Enforcement and Customs and Border Protection frequently violate these standards. In 2018, for example, 2,094 pregnant women were held in immigration detention (Cerón-Becerra 2022). Even prior to the pandemic, pregnant women held in immigration detention were often forced to birth alone. In many instances, they may not even know the whereabouts of partners being held in different detention facilities. A CNM described the emotional toll of this separation: "One patient in particular, she cried every visit, asking, 'How is my husband going to know? He doesn't even know where I am. Where is he? I haven't seen him in so long.' And there was a lot of crying from her. I was in the hospital one day, and they called me to come talk to her because she was just crying, crying, crying. And you just had to unfortunately say, 'No, we are just unable to contact him, and he will not be able to come.'"

Nurses and CNMs described numerous other misgivings over how hospital, prison, and immigration policies were causing harm to their patients, especially at the height of the pandemic. Yet, they often felt unable to provide a more empowering context for the birth. Many, however, described the ways they tried to offer compassion to patients in vulnerable circumstances through practices such as stocking patients with extra supplies, including diapers and formula, and trying to be more present when other support people could not be there. Such efforts may have been more concerted among CNMs and nurses than OB-GYNs, given the different paradigms of care.

Experiences of Care as the Pandemic Evolved

Jazmine's, Anessa's, Lina's, and Camila's narratives illustrate the range of experiences that women had while seeking prenatal care and giving birth during the pandemic. While using a midwife often contributed to more positive experiences, other institutional factors and provider inconsistencies at times created situations that they described as negligent or disempowering. Women's social positions also played a significant role in their overall experiences of care.

Jazmine: Perceptions of Midwifery Care

When Jazmine began prenatal care during her first of three pregnancies in 2018, the receptionist scheduled her with a midwife. She is unsure why her first appointment was with a midwife, but it is perhaps because Texas Tech often diverts low-risk pregnancies covered by Medicaid to midwifery care. At the time, Jazmine was not aware there was a difference between midwives and OB-GYNs. However, her first appointment with a midwife went far better than any medical encounter she had previously had with an OB-GYN. After that, she sought care through midwives for all her pregnancies.

Of her experiences with midwives, Jazmine said, "They are a little more personal, more open to listening to my problems. They're just a little gentler when it comes to the birthing process." During the first birth, Jazmine described what could have felt like a traumatic experience due to a retained placenta. If the placenta does not come out entirely after the birth, it can cause severe infection and hemorrhaging. To avoid these complications, a midwife or OB-GYN will manually remove the placenta, a process that women sometimes describe as more painful than the birth itself. Following the manual removal of the placenta, Jazmine hemorrhaged severely enough to need a blood transfusion and infusions of iron to manage the anemia that followed so much blood loss. While she described the manual placenta removal as excruciatingly painful, she felt her midwife treated her with care and clearly explained everything, helping her to feel calm about what was happening.

For her second pregnancy, her first appointment was with an OB-GYN. After a disappointing and rushed visit with poor communication, she insisted on scheduling her subsequent visits with a midwife. Although there was not a midwife on call at the time of birth, a resident who had trained under the midwives attended the birth. Jazmine said, "The doctor I got was equally amazing [as the midwives]." By her third pregnancy, Jazmine knew to request a midwife when she called to make her first appointment. Again, she described a positive birth experience.

While Jazmine described overwhelmingly positive experiences in her clinical encounters with midwives, there are ways her care fell short and put her health at risk. In particular, Jazmine experienced limitations in the scope and duration of care because of how structural factors exacerbated by the pandemic impeded her access to follow-up care. Between the birth of her second child in June 2020 and her third pregnancy less than a year later, Jazmine expressed a desire for various forms of care that she perceived to be out of reach. She knew she was struggling with postpartum depression but felt too ill and overwhelmed to schedule her postpartum visit before the expiration date that appeared on her Medicaid paperwork. As explained in chapter 1, her Medicaid should have continued through the duration of the public health emergency, yet Jazmin was unaware of this. Had she gone to a postpartum visit, it is possible that her midwife would have referred her to services to treat her postpartum depression. Perhaps she may have also learned that she could still access birth control through her continued Medicaid coverage, given her desire to avoid another pregnancy.

Between her second and third pregnancies, Jazmine's family was also struggling economically. Jazmine had left work to stay with the children, reducing their household income. Financially, it did not make sense for them to pay for childcare for multiple children with the low wages she had been earning. Her husband, Luis, was working at Walmart, but he did not make enough to support their growing family. Even with the assistance they received through food stamps and public housing, they often did not have enough money to buy groceries and had to borrow money from Luis's parents. Although the couple wanted to prioritize eating healthy, they could often only afford cheap, frozen food and cans of tuna.

In these circumstances of barely getting by, Luis learned of an opportunity to take a much higher-paying job that would put him on the road for weeks at a time. Taking the job would mean Luis would be gone for long stretches of time, possibly missing the birth of their third child, but it would alleviate their financial struggles. The couple decided to make the situation as short-term as possible, as Luis would continue looking for work locally. Yet, a year into this arrangement, Luis continued working out-of-town. Jazmine said, "People are like, 'Everyone is hiring.' Yeah, everyone who is just gonna give you minimum wage and crap hours. We have three kids and need something a little more stable." Before the birth, Jazmine was worried Luis might not even be present when she went into labor. Although the new job paid better, it still did not come with any paid leave. When the couple received their tax returns, they were relieved to have extra money through the Child Tax Credit, which the American Rescue Plan had temporarily increased. This extra money enabled Luis to take a month off work so that he could be present in the weeks leading up to the birth.

The birth went quickly, without complications. Again, Jazmine described the care she received from her midwife in positive terms. Jazmine was unaware, however, that numerous midwives had left the practice throughout the pandemic. The departure of midwives in part reflects a larger pattern in shortages of health care providers as the pandemic exacerbated burnout and created untenable work environments. In mid-2021, the World Health Organization reported a global shortage of nearly one million midwives. By the time Jazmine scheduled her postpartum visit, the midwifery practice was down to a single midwife. When she missed her appointment after misplacing her wallet, she was unable to schedule another appointment prior to the date when she believed her Medicaid expired. She had been determined to go to her postpartum visit this time given her history of postpartum depression and a strong desire for birth control. When she could not schedule an appointment with a midwife, she traveled to Juárez to obtain birth control.

Jazmine's experiences reflect that simply having midwives available is not enough to ensure optimal care, especially given the structural constraints women may be experiencing. While having a midwife made for positive clinical encounters, even getting into an appointment to have these encounters was rife with challenges. Institutional constraints further posed limitations on access to midwifery care, as a once thriving midwifery practice took a significant hit during the pandemic. It is important to consider that although Jazmine had economic struggles, other aspects of her positionality served as protective factors. Significantly, Jazmine emphasized the benefits conferred by her US citizenship. Her mother and older sister had been undocumented throughout her childhood, so she intimately understood the ways immigration status can exclude a person from health services. It was her US citizenship that enabled her to obtain Medicaid. Additionally, she maintained strong cross-border ties to family members living in Juárez, which facilitated her access to private practices in Mexico when she was unable to receive the care she needed in the United States.

Anessa: Provider Inconsistencies and Communication Failures

Anessa began feeling contractions at around 8:00 a.m. one morning in January 2021, during the peak of the first Omicron wave. By noon, her contractions were still about ten minutes apart. She knew that she still had awhile before the delivery, but it was her first pregnancy and she was nervous, so she decided to go to the hospital. Although she had received her prenatal care through the CNMs, there was not a midwife on call in labor and delivery that day. Instead, a resident who had likely trained under the CNMs attended to her. The resident gave Anessa an ultrasound and told her she could wait to see how things progressed. By 6:00 pm, the resident suggested Anessa go home and return when the contractions were stronger and closer together. At the advice of the resident, Anessa also went for a long walk. Walking can naturally augment labor by promoting a position that helps the baby drop down in the pelvis. When providers recommend walking, it can reduce the reliance on inducing labor (Shojaei et al. 2021). The walk seems to have helped Anessa, as she returned to the hospital three hours later with contractions that were two minutes apart.

When Anessa returned to the hospital, the earlier resident had left, and she instead saw the attending physician. According to Anessa, the attending physician informed her that the earlier ultrasound showed that the baby was not breathing and that she should have stayed at the hospital to be induced. Babies do not technically breath while in utero. Rather, fetal breathing movements, also called practice breaths, move amniotic fluid in and out of the lungs. The movement strengthens lungs and helps prepare the baby to take their first real breaths after birth. While the presence of these movements is a sign of a healthy fetus, it is completely normal for babies to go long stretches without making any. In fact, fetal breathing movements are often absent at the onset of labor and their absence can be used as one indication that a person is in true labor as opposed to false labor (Boylan, O'Donovan, and Owens 1985). Different providers have varying views on whether or not to admit a patient if labor has started but is progressing slowly. Many OB-GYNs prefer to admit a patient and augment labor with Pitocin, a synthetic version of oxytocin that is used to stimulate contractions. Midwives and physicians who have been influenced by the midwifery model may be less inclined to rely on technological intervention in favor of promoting natural methods to stimulate labor, such as going for a long walk.

It seems that no one explained these nuances to Anessa, or at least, no one explained in a way she understood. Instead, she had the impression that her baby was not breathing and at risk of dying. She immediately became anxious and fearful that the resident had been negligent. She said, "After they told me this, I began to sob. It angered me that they hadn't told me anything. Since so much time had passed, I thought my baby was going to die."

When Anessa, still crying, asked why they had told her to leave, the nurse simply told her, "You are going to be fine. We will check you. Everything will be OK." Anessa said, "But I felt so powerless. After that, I didn't have any faith in them." It is likely that Anessa really did not need to fear for the baby's life. Yet, the clashing approaches of the providers who attended to her and a lack of communication regarding the medical situation at hand led a normal occurrence during labor to feel overwhelmingly tragic for Anessa.

It is possible that language barriers factored into the poor communication. A majority of people in El Paso are bilingual to some degree but are not necessarily able to communicate effectively in both languages. It can also be easy to misread a person's degree of fluency in either language. My conversations with Anessa were exclusively in Spanish, although she did report she spoke some English. Among physicians who are not fluent in Spanish, there is a tendency to rely on other medical support personnel, such as nurses, to translate. Anessa's questioning of her nurse suggests she felt better able to communicate with the nurse, yet this nurse may not have had a detailed enough understanding of the situation to fully explain everything to Anessa in a way that could have put her at ease.

Further complicating matters was the fact that Anessa tested positive for COVID-19 upon admission to labor and delivery. At the time, the hospital required testing only upon admission, but not during her earlier visit. Although she was asymptomatic, the COVID-19 diagnosis further compounded Anessa's fears, as she began to worry she would be separated from the baby. A nurse assured her the baby could stay in the room with her as long as they all remained masked. However, if the baby required a transfer to the NICU, neither Anessa nor her husband would be able to enter. Given Anessa's impression that the baby was not properly breathing, she had very real fears that the baby would have to go to the NICU alone.

Fortunately, Anessa described the birth itself in more positive terms. Upon admission, she quickly accepted the epidural offered to her as planned. She described the epidural as making the contractions tolerable and the rest of the labor easier. Once her cervix fully dilated, the doctor and nurse coached her on how to push. Her daughter came quickly and let out cries with her first gasps of air.

Anessa's experience shows how a lack of continuity of providers contributed to experiences of anguish and trauma during labor. Having providers with different paradigms of what constitutes optimal care created conflicting messages for Anessa, and there was a subsequent lack of communication about her providers' interpretations of normal processes. Although Anessa described positive interactions with her midwives during her prenatal visits, the shortage of midwives within the overall practice resulted in a shift in approaches to care during her labor. Thus, institutional factors may constrain the potential for a midwifery model to contribute to more positive birth experiences.

Challenges in continuity of care continued for Anessa postpartum. Her only postpartum checkup was automatically scheduled with the attending physician for the birth, even though all her prenatal care had been with the midwives. As described earlier, Anessa was experiencing severe mastitis and postpartum depression at the time of this visit. She received a referral to the emergency room for the mastitis, but the hospital turned her away because CHIP Perinatal would not cover the services. The fact that she had CHIP Perinatal was a result of her precarious immigration status. She received no referral or follow-up for her postpartum depression. Perhaps if Anessa's visit had been with a provider more familiar with her situation, she may have received additional information on community clinics and the hospital discount program in order to help her access the postpartum services she desperately needed.

Lina: Finding Compassionate Care for High-Risk Situations

"When I started this journey, when I found out I was pregnant, I was like, 'I don't want a medicated labor.' My sister was laughing at me because she said I was a hippy. But I wanted everything natural." In line with these desires, Lina initially sought prenatal care with midwives in San Antonio, which is where she was living when she became pregnant. What also drove Lina to midwifery was her negative perception of doctors. As an occupational therapist assistant, she was constantly around physicians. She said, "I have to deal with a lot of doctors. I don't know what it is about doctors, but most of them are really, really cold. They don't really care. I thought I was going to encounter that, so that's why I didn't want to go with a doctor."

Lina did, however, have to transition from seeing midwives to an OB-GYN when her ultrasound showed fetal abnormalities and the care would be beyond the scope of what midwives can provide. Lina's first interaction with a high-risk OB-GYN in San Antonio went terribly. He provided very little information about the enlarged ventricles on the fetus's brain that had appeared on the twenty-week anatomy scan and immediately encouraged Lina to terminate the pregnancy. This encounter reflects what sociologist Angela Frederick (2017) describes as a "normalcy project" in which providers seek to manage risk and prevent disability without consideration of the mother's own positionality and feelings over possibly having a child with a disability. The doctor went on to encourage Lina to make a quick decision. If she wanted to have the procedure in Texas, she only had eight days to decide. Otherwise, she would have to travel out of state. At the time, in early 2021, Lina could have terminated the pregnancy in Texas for fetal abnormalities up to twenty-two weeks' gestation. At the time of writing, she would have never had the option to have an abortion in Texas. Ultimately, Lina left the appointment in confusion and despair over an unclear diagnosis.

Lina initially decided to have an abortion. However, she was unable to get an appointment in San Antonio before the cutoff date of when she could legally have the procedure in Texas. Instead, she scheduled an appointment in New Mexico. She was packing her bags for the trip when she decided she would continue with the pregnancy. With a still unclear diagnosis and strong religious faith, she was looking for a sign for what she should do. She interpreted her inability to get an appointment locally as the sign she needed. Her and her husband continued packing though. If they were going to have the baby, they knew they would need family support. They both quit their stable jobs that had offered them a comfortable income and relocated to live with Lina's parents in El Paso.

In El Paso, Lina resumed care with a high-risk OB-GYN. In leaving her job, she had lost her health insurance, so she applied for Medicaid for Pregnant Women. This combination of factors made her nervous about the care she would receive, given her negative perceptions of doctors and the added worry that medical staff would judge and treat her differently for having Medicaid. However, she described her high-risk OB-GYN in El Paso as completely different from what she had expected, saying, "She's been nothing but amazing, honestly." Lina was also relieved to discover that Medicaid fully covered the specialist visits and extra exams, whereas she would have had high out-of-pocket expenses with her private insurance.

As she neared the end of the pregnancy, Lina had accepted the fact that the birth was not going to go the way she had first imagined. To her surprise, her OB-GYN was supportive of avoiding a C-section as long as there did not appear to be increasing amounts of fluid in the baby's brain. However, the birth would require coordination with the pediatric neurosurgeon, who was pushing for a C-section to control the timing of the birth to align with his schedule. In the end, Lina's OB-GYN successfully pushed back against a planned C-section, although Lina was induced at thirty-seven weeks' gestation due to preeclampsia.

While Lina had prepared herself for a high intervention birth, she felt disempowered by the way providers treated her at various points during and after the labor. She continued feeling strong emotions about the birth in the months that followed. With the induction, it took over two days for labor to progress and she was at the hospital for a total of four days. During that time, she described "fighting for my rights," saying, "Everybody's telling me what to do and how to do it. Nobody's listening to me. In the delivery room, there were like twenty people in there. There were like fourteen different specialists. I had him for two minutes, and everybody's like, 'OK, well, we're going to the NICU.' So everybody started walking away, and I'm left with so many questions." Unable to even move around yet, Lina felt abandoned, but she sent her husband to be with the baby. Since he could not use a phone in the NICU, Lina received no updates about the baby's status. It was four hours before Lina recovered enough mobility to go to the NICU to hold her baby.

Lina's narrative reflects a number of key issues related to the challenges of finding compassionate care. First, the label of *high risk* immediately limits a person's options for providers. She was automatically ineligible for care with a midwife, which had been her plan. Many hospitals have only one high-risk provider; if there is not one, the patient receives a referral for care elsewhere.[7] For Lina, this meant she had extremely limited choices in terms of who she saw. In San Antonio, she felt traumatized by the high-risk OB-GYN. While she felt supported by the high-risk OB-GYN in El Paso, her care involved multiple specialists. During the labor and delivery, Lina felt disempowered by the degree of physician coordination and control over the birth. While Lina rationalized that this structure was for the sake of the baby, she still felt abandoned at a time of vulnerability. Given the circumstances of the pandemic, there were additional levels of uncertainty that could have potentially made the situation far worse. For example, if Lina had tested positive for COVID-19, she would not have been able to visit the baby in the NICU.

Lina's social position enabled her to have various options available, including being able to make a decision about whether to terminate the pregnancy and being able to relocate to a different city. As a US-born citizen, Lina could travel through the internal border checkpoints on the way Albuquerque, New Mexico. Her and her husband both had stable employment prior to the pregnancy, enabling them to have some savings available for emergencies. Having grown up in Juárez in a relatively privileged family that owned a business, Lina also felt at ease travelling to Mexico for care if she was unable to get the services she needed in the United States.

Camila: Complex Prenatal Care during Early Pandemic Lockdown

In early April 2020, Camila arrived for her full anatomy scan appointment at twenty-three weeks' gestation. While this sonogram typically occurs at twenty weeks' gestation, initial pandemic lockdowns had gone into effect just weeks earlier, leading to a delay in her appointment. Camila was feeling excited to see the baby. The pregnancy had been a welcome surprise for Camila, who for years had thought health issues would prevent her from ever being able to conceive. Clouding her excitement was the fact that her mother would not be able to join her due to the new pandemic regulations barring visitors. Given that the baby's father had decided he did not want to be involved, Camila's mother, along with her father, brother, and aunt, had stepped into roles as surrogate parents.

In the sonogram room, the atmosphere quickly turned tense and then frightening. The baby's heart rate had registered at almost 300 beats per minute (bpm). Anything over 180 bpm is concerning, as a sign of tachycardia. The high heart rate that characterizes tachycardia is an indication that the heart is only having shallow contractions that are not forceful enough to pump sufficient blood, which can ultimately lead to heart failure. Later, doctors would confirm that multiple holes in the baby's heart were causing the tachycardia. The pediatric cardiologist who spoke with Camila told her that it would be the last day of her pregnancy. She would either lose the baby or require medical transport to Houston or San Antonio to deliver. Given the pandemic, Camila would have to go alone.

Before making a decision about transporting Camila, her doctors wanted to see if they could stabilize the baby's heart with medication. As the medications did in fact begin to work, the medical team decided they could wait to see how things progressed. From that point forward, Camila said, "day-by-day, I didn't know if I was going to deliver." For the subsequent two weeks, Camila remained in the Cardiovascular Intensive Care Unit for monitoring and establishing a regime for cardiovascular medications. For those two weeks, Camila was alone in her hospital room, not permitted any visitors due to pandemic restrictions.

During the hospitalization, Camila went off the medications she had long taken to manage post-traumatic stress disorder, major depression, and generalized anxiety. Initially, her doctors wanted her off the medication while they calibrated the dosages of the heart medication. Camila asked that her cardiologist and OB-GYN communicate this information with her psychiatrist. Her psychiatrist was, after all, located in the same medical complex. Her medical team assured her that they had sent him a message, although later medical encounters would reveal that the psychiatrist had never received this message. When Camila did not hear anything back from her psychiatrist, she decided to stay off her previous medications. She had already stopped taking them for two weeks while hospitalized and she had lingering concerns that it was the medications that had caused her baby's heart problem.

Once the baby's status stabilized, Camila was able to return home. She would have multiple visits with specialists on a weekly basis. Initially, Camila felt relief and hope that her baby would be healthy. Yet, her fears for the baby combined with having stopped her medications spiraled. On multiple occasions, Camila went to the emergency room with symptoms of panic attacks and suicidal thoughts. On a routine visit for bloodwork, she was not feeling well and felt like no one had been listening to her. Frustrated, she left and walked upstairs to labor and delivery. There, she encountered providers whom she knew from previous visits. This was also the first time she had follow-up with her psychiatrist. Finally, the fetal cardiologist and psychiatrist coordinated a plan for care. This was the first time Camila received follow-up on her own medications and what she could take alongside the baby's medications. She expressed her frustration over the previous lack of communication, saying, "When I stopped taking my medications, since day one, I told them, 'My psychiatrist is here. Like, two minutes walking. Can you tell him what is going on? I need to know if this is OK.' Nobody ever told him. Nobody ever got the importance or thought it was important until way later." For the final month of pregnancy, Camila finally started feeling better.

The birth again involved instances when Camila felt like her providers were not listening to her nor coordinating with each other. As soon as Camila reached full-term at thirty-seven weeks' gestation, she was induced. Her mother joined her as her birth companion. Induction can be a long process, as it bypasses the pregnant person's hormonal signaling that prepares the body for labor and birth. Given that slow or stalled progression of labor may result in a C-section, individual providers may engage in various strategies to speed up the induction process. When Camila's contractions first started, she was not feeling much discomfort. Her nurse informed her that if the contractions did not hurt, then labor would not progress. This nurse kept upping the dosage of Pitocin, the medication used to induce and augment labor, even after a doctor had instructed the nurse to keep the dose low so that Camila would not exhaust herself with contractions before her cervix had dilated. Despite the doctor's instructions, the nurse continued to increase the Pitocin dosage without Camila's consent. Although Camila had wanted to avoid an epidural, she ended up requesting one. Pitocin, especially when used more aggressively, typically causes more painful contractions than if labor had progressed without augmentation.

Camila also described interactions with two OB-GYNs over the course of her induction. One explained everything that was happening and sought Camila's consent for exams and procedures. The other OB-GYN left Camila feeling violated when he stripped her membranes without informing her beforehand. This procedure is one mechanism for stimulating labor. Camila described the stripping of membranes as, "The most painful thing that has ever happened to me." Having the procedure take place without warning further made it feel traumatic. Fortunately, Camila felt well supported by a different OB-GYN when it came time to deliver.

Like Lina, Camila had prepared herself for a NICU transfer immediately following the birth. She held her baby for one minute before they took him. Hospital staff had initially told her that her mother would be able to accompany the baby to the NICU until she recovered enough to go herself. Instead, the NICU denied her mother entry because she was not a parent of the baby. Luckily, the baby did not have to stay there long, and they were able to go home together within seventy-two hours.

The effects of being at the hospital continued, however. Camila and her family returned home on a Friday. By Monday, they all tested positive for COVID-19. As Camila had tested negative upon admission to the hospital, it seems likely they contracted COVID-19 at the hospital. Although the baby was asymptomatic and Camila and her mother had only mild symptoms, at the time, COVID-19 was still so new that Camila felt panic. She said, "I didn't know anybody that had COVID at that time that had survived. It was like, they have COVID and they pass away. When my mom told me she was positive, I was bawling. I cried so much. In my mind, I was like, 'She's gonna die.'"

Throughout her narrative, Camila reflected on both positive and negative experiences she had with her providers. While she spoke highly of some individual providers, she ultimately found a lack of coordination and inconsistency with providers as having negative ramifications for her health. Additionally, there were instances when providers left her feeling ignored. The circumstances of the pandemic exacerbated these negative experiences, as the pandemic limited the crucial support she could receive from family members, especially during her two-week hospitalization. Constantly changing policies may have also contributed to the poor communication over whether Camila's mother could enter the NICU.

Implications for Achieving Birth Justice

The clinical experiences women described show both the possibilities and limitations for ensuring compassionate care in uncertain and precarious circumstances. For many women, having access to compassionate and structurally competent providers helped mitigate the structural vulnerabilities that contribute to maternal harm. Brisa and Jazmine both emphasized how the care they received from their midwives contributed to positive memories of their births, despite events that could have easily contributed to birth trauma. This is in large part because midwifery training focuses on humanizing the birth experience, rather than pathologizing birth. This is not to say that OB-GYNs cannot also provide compassionate care. However, the enculturation and training involved in becoming a physician can contribute to a dehumanized approach to care (Haque and Waytz 2012). Lina's, Anessa's, and Camila's experiences reflect the unevenness in how individual physicians approach care and interact with patients. Lina and Camila in particular had positive experiences with some OB-GYNs but extremely negative experiences with others.

While women using midwifery care often spoke very highly of their clinical encounters with their midwives, there were never enough midwives within the Texas Tech/UMC system to ensure that midwifery care could always be accessible for those who desired it. For Anessa, this led to inconsistent approaches to her care. Combined with poor communication, this led Anessa to feel traumatized by a benign situation. The midwifery shortage also interrupted Jazmine's ability to receive follow-up care. The exhausting working conditions of the pandemic had further exacerbated institutional challenges in retaining midwives.

Beyond OB-GYNs and midwives, different types of health care workers shape experiences of care. Camila in particular felt disempowered and harmed by the way a nurse treated her while in labor. Contrasting the experiences of Brisa and Anessa shows how hospital staff, such as those in billing and patient services, can serve as gatekeepers to services. The resulting institutional interactions can contribute to different patient experiences and outcomes, even at the same hospital. While Brisa immediately received information on payment plans and applying for the hospital discount program, Anessa received no such information during her emergency room visit with severe mastitis. Their experiences show the significance of fostering structural competency at all levels.

While access to compassionate providers is an important component of achieving birth justice, it is only a piece of the puzzle. The quality of providers does not matter if people cannot access them. Both Brisa and Anessa had negative clinical encounters that they tied to their exclusion from health services that were beyond the scope of their CHIP Perinatal coverage. Jazmine's perceived exclusion from services postpartum also limited her ability to receive the care that she needed. Beyond that, the confines of care during pregnancy and birth cannot remedy the structural constraints that women experience in their everyday lives. The fact that some women experienced multiple forms of maternal harm, despite reporting positive clinical experiences, shows the importance of going beyond obstetric violence as an analytical tool and engaging with the policies and social contexts that produce reproductive violence outside of the clinical context.

6

Navigating *Impotencia* during the Postpartum Period

In September of 2020, Itzel, her boyfriend, and her oldest of three daughters from a previous relationship tested positive for COVID-19. During their isolation, Itzel's period was late. A home pregnancy test came back positive. Neither Itzel nor her boyfriend had wanted a child together, and Itzel had used various forms of birth control to avoid pregnancy. At one point, she was hopeful an IUD would be an easy option, but after having it removed due to persistent, severe pain, she began taking birth control pills instead. She was still on the pill when she became pregnant.

Itzel believes the combination of their COVID-19 isolation and the unplanned pregnancy led her boyfriend to leave her during the first trimester. When I last spoke to Iztel three months after the birth, she had yet to hear from him again. As a single mother of four children, including a newborn, Itzel faced a number of struggles during the postpartum period while the pandemic continued.

Among Itzel's dilemmas was deciding whether to return to work following the birth. Just before her pregnancy, she had started a new job as a secretary for a construction company. The position involved a slight pay cut and she lost the sick leave she had accumulated at her previous job, but it came with shorter hours that enabled her to pick her children up from school as opposed to sending them to an afterschool program. Had she remained at her old job, she could have taken up to twelve-weeks of unpaid leave following the birth in accordance with the Family and Medical Leave Act (FMLA). She could have also used her sick leave in order to receive pay during some of this time. Since she had been with a new company for less than a year, she had no legal rights under FMLA. Instead, her supervisor told her she could have three weeks off following the birth. Itzel also believed she would likely not qualify for unemployment benefits if she did not return to work following the birth. Although the Pandemic Unemployment Assistance (PUA) program temporarily expanded benefits to caretakers who could not seek work due to school and childcare closures, the birth occurred after area schools had reopened. Technically, Itzel had access to childcare. However, she was terrified of putting a newborn in daycare during a pandemic.

While still pregnant, Itzel felt conflicted about what to do after the birth. She needed money to support her children, especially since she would not be able to count on child support from the baby's father, who had disappeared. She also did not want to rely on government assistance. An indication of her hesitancy to use publicly funded programs was that a month prior to the birth, she had still not applied for WIC, even though she knew she would qualify and had used the program in the past. For the time being, she felt like the food stamps she received were sufficient support and she was worried she would be using resources that someone else might need more than her.

After the birth, Itzel decided she could not go back to work three weeks postpartum. Fearful of the health consequences of putting her newborn in daycare, she quit her job. Jobless and abandoned by the baby's father, she pieced together child support from the father of her older children, checks from the temporarily expanded Child Tax Credit,[1] food stamps, WIC, and rental assistance. This was not an ideal situation for her, given her desire to generate a stable income. Additionally, she spent a significant amount of time submitting paperwork for various programs. The rental assistance program, for example, required her to reapply every two months.

The extended border closure further complicated Itzel's potential for having a safer childcare arrangement. In the past, Itzel's mother would regularly cross the border from Juárez to help care for her grandchildren, which had facilitated Itzel's return to work following the births of her previous children. However, Itzel's mother was not a US citizen and only had a border crossing card, which she could not use to enter the United States while the border remained closed for nonessential travel. Had Itzel had family support available, she would have felt comfortable leaving the baby with family, saying, "They [my family] would take the necessary precautions to not put the baby at risk. In a daycare, obviously it is difficult because they have many employees."

Alternatively, some US citizens and residents regularly cross to Mexico to have family members care for their children. While Itzel is a US citizen, she was unable to cross the border with ease. This is because her citizenship had been put into question, likely due to the circumstances of her birth. In 1992, Itzel's parents had used their border crossing cards to come to El Paso for the birth in a free-standing birth center run by midwives. In an unequal border context, cross-border births are a practice that ensures US citizenship to the child alongside the symbolic and tangible benefits this citizenship entails. Given that Itzel's parents would be paying for health services in full, as opposed to having insurance offset the costs, a free-standing birth center was a more affordable option than a hospital.

When Itzel was entering adulthood, she decided to relocate to El Paso. When she applied for her US passport, however, the US State Department denied her application. Itzel was at a loss, as she knew she was born in the United States, had a Texas birth certificate, and had secured other US identity documents. Her inability to secure a US passport reflects a larger pattern of passport denials to Latino border residents who had a midwife-attended birth. From the 1960s through early 2000s, there is evidence that midwives in Texas border counties falsely registered some births as taking place in the United States. Those cases have served as a pretext to question the citizenship of thousands of US-born citizens who were delivered outside of a hospital setting by a midwife (Sieff 2018). Often, rather than issuing a straightforward denial, the State Department asks applicants to produce additional evidence of the circumstances of the birth. This may prove to be an impossible task.

After her passport denial, Itzel used her Texas driver's license to enter the United States, which is an acceptable means of entering by land for a US citizen. Yet, she feared that repeated crossings without a passport could lead to further investigations by Border Patrol, denial of her entry, and separation from her children. She was especially concerned about what might happen during the Donald Trump administration. As a result, she had not returned to Mexico in ten years. Itzel had consulted with various lawyers about the issue. Some lawyers said they would not even take the case. Given the common practice of borrowing identity documents among immigrant networks (Horton 2016), they may have been skeptical of Itzel's claim to citizenship. A lawyer who did agree to take her case told her it would cost $10,000—a sum of money she did not have. Itzel explained her fears resulting from this situation: "I'm always fearful that one day they are going to say to me that I can't use my ID, that I can't use my social security. It will be this way until I get a lawyer, so I'm always scared that something could happen. When you know that you were born here. That you are not lying. That is what I think gives you the most *impotencia* [powerlessness], that you know you are telling the truth, but unfortunately, you don't have the means to hire a lawyer. So there is not much you can do."

For people with young children and infants, like Itzel, the pandemic created impossible dilemmas over managing childcare and work. Single parents such as Itzel often more profoundly felt this dilemma, lacking the support of a partner with whom to share the labor of childcare and to contribute economically to the household. While family may help mitigate some of these challenges, in Itzel's case, the border closure cut her off from potentially important familial help, especially childcare. Throughout her narrative, Itzel evoked the term *impotencia* to describe how she felt about the context of her life. This sense of powerlessness fundamentally affected her decisions about how to best care for her family, and each possible option could have devastating outcomes.

Itzel and other women were forced to navigate constraining circumstances during the postpartum period as the pandemic persisted. For many, crises that emerged in the earlier phases of the pandemic continued to reverberate in ways that left them feeling like they had no good options, with continued experiences of conjugated harm. Yet, as Jessica Cerdeña (2023) also shows through her research on immigrant mothers during the pandemic, women pushed onward. In pushing onward, women exercised their agency in spite of inhibiting circumstances. While women actively made decisions about returning to work, managing childcare, and navigating economic crises, disempowering circumstances framed their options. Thus, the actions women took in pushing onward often came with consequences that imposed a toll on their physical and emotional well-being.

Postpartum Struggles in the Border Context

The pandemic precipitated what became the deepest economic recession of the post–World War II era. However, the economic recovery occurred more quickly than initially predicted, at least on a national scale (Center on Budget and Policy Priorities 2023). Like the initial shock of the pandemic, the recovery has been uneven. A person's social status, geographic location, and how much they lost—economically, socially, and physically—contributed to their ability to rebound as the pandemic subsided.

The continued economic reverberations of the pandemic were especially pronounced in US border cities that are dependent upon cross-border economic activities. In El Paso, prior to the pandemic, 30 percent of retail sales were from Mexican shoppers. The nineteen-month border closure that lasted until November 2021 halted the pattern of crossing regularly for shopping and leisure, significantly disrupting the border economy and contributing to job losses.

Nationally, pandemic job losses were highest among low-income women of color. Nearly one year into the pandemic, 8 percent of women reported quitting their job for a pandemic-related reason, but this figure was substantially higher for Black and Latina women and low-income workers, and 17 percent of women with incomes less than 200 percent of the federal poverty level (FPL) had left work (Ranji et al. 2021). While federal supplements to unemployment benefits helped offset the economic repercussions of job losses, especially in geographic locations with a lower cost of living such as El Paso (Cañas, Orrenius, and Coia 2022), many of the women we interviewed did not qualify for unemployment, or at least they did not think they did. Itzel, for example, had resigned over her inability to return to work three weeks postpartum. Since she resigned, as opposed to waiting for her employer to fire her when she did not return to work quickly enough, she believed she did not qualify for unemployment. Although federal stipulations allow for unemployment if a person quits for a good cause, states have different interpretations of this clause. In Texas, stipulations state that a person maintains eligibility for unemployment if they quit to care for a minor child who has a medical illness. Fear that a newborn would be subjected to medical illness is not sufficient cause.

Like Itzel, many women who left the workforce were balancing the demands of childcare and virtual schooling with their decisions about work. Schools reopening may have somewhat alleviated childcare challenges for parents of older children, but insecurities persisted for families with young children and newborns. Further, the early pandemic led to widespread temporary closures of childcare facilities, and some of these centers never recovered. Two years into the pandemic, 8 percent of childcare facilities in Texas had not reopened and the *Texas Tribune* classified El Paso County as a childcare desert, having 3.2 times as many children as spots available in registered childcare facilities (Hernandez and Huang 2022). Of course, this figure fails to capture the informal means of childcare that people rely on, some of which depends upon crossing the US-Mexico border. Many women we interviewed had family members who took care of their children. In my own case, when my son was four months old, my husband and I had to return to work. Not ready to put him in daycare and risk potential exposure to COVID-19, my mother-in-law travelled from Bolivia to help with childcare for six months. When she left, we then took my son to a woman who cared for two or three children at a time out of her home. This was an informal, unregistered childcare situation, not accounted for in statistics of registered daycares. While such practices are common in the region, the border closure significantly disrupted usual patterns. Grandparents, nannies, and other caretakers who reside in Juárez were no longer able to cross if they did not have US citizenship or permanent residency. The border closure made strikingly clear that El Paso depends upon the labor of people residing in Juárez.

Even after the border reopened, economic struggles persisted as inflation reduced household purchasing power. In the midst of increasing prices for basic necessities, there was a national formula shortage that began when the primary production facility for Abbott Nutrition halted production of infant formula in February 2022. This decision came after medical investigations linked two deaths and four severe illnesses of infants to a rare strain of bacteria found in Abbott's production facility in Michigan. A whistleblower report pointed to widespread negligence within the factory. The lack of oversight by regulatory bodies such as the Food and Drug Administration during the pandemic had contributed to this negligence. Given that Abbott controls a significant share of the formula market in the United States and was the primary supplier for WIC and other nutritional programs in a majority of US states, the halted production led to a widespread and prolonged shortage. The insufficient supply led the Joe Biden administration to airlift formula from other countries while other formula makers increased production capacities (Angrist 2022).

During the earliest months of the formula shortage, Texas was among the states with an out-of-stock rate greater than 50 percent, meaning over half of all formula products were unavailable in a given period (Pathak, Jarsulic, and Ahmed 2022). The border context to some extent alleviated the effects of limited supplies in El Paso. As the formula shortage was limited to the US market, stores in Mexico remained stocked. Although Mexican stores are unable to accept WIC benefits, the cost of formula is roughly half of the price in Mexico compared to the US. Based on our interviews and in monitoring Facebook groups for finding formula, it appears that people could generally find a basic formula product and that the primary struggle was finding specialty formulas, such as those required by babies born preterm or with specific nutritional needs.

Conflicts in Returning to Work, Childcare, and Persistent Economic Crises

For many women, hardships generated during earlier stages of the pandemic reverberated throughout the postpartum period and shaped their decisions about childcare, returning to work, and even marriage. In many instances, women felt like they had no good options, as any decision could result in negative ramifications in other aspects of their lives. As a result, their postpartum experiences were often rife with social, emotional, and economic struggles.

Accepting Lower Pay to Minimize Health Risks

Eliana gave birth to her first child in early summer of 2021. While pregnant, she felt ambivalent about parenthood. At thirty-six years old and not in a serious relationship, she enjoyed her independence and had thought that perhaps she would never have a child. When she discovered she was pregnant following a fling with a man who was in another relationship, she was initially uncertain about whether to continue with the pregnancy. In continuing with the pregnancy, she also decided she would not depend on any support from the father, choosing to leave his name off her daughter's birth certificate and not seek child support.

While Eliana did not have financial or affective support from the father, she did have her parents who provided various sources of help following the birth, including childcare so that she could return to work without leaving the baby in daycare. However, the circumstances of the pandemic dictated what type of jobs she felt safe accepting. Just before her pregnancy, Eliana had completed her associate's degree and licensure to become an occupational therapist assistant. For years, she had worked in a low-paying job without benefits as a home health aide, tending to elderly clients. Initially, she was excited about the prospect of a higher-paying job with benefits thanks to her new degree. However, becoming pregnant and having a newborn during the pandemic made Eliana pause in seeking a new, higher-paying job. The jobs in her new field of work would be in contexts with high risks of exposure to COVID-19. Throughout her pregnancy and first year postpartum, she continued working at her lower-paying job in an effort to protect her daughter. While her job offered her parental leave, it would be unpaid. She saved her stimulus checks that were a part of the CARES Act in order to take time off. After eight weeks of unpaid leave following the birth, she needed and desperately wanted more time with her daughter, but financial concerns forced her to return to work. She said, "I returned to work with literally zero dollars in my bank account." She had also put her car payments on hold and was fearful she may lose the vehicle she depended upon for travel to clients' homes.

A key factor that facilitated Eliana's return to work was the fact that she could rely on her parents for childcare. Like Itzel, Eliana felt that leaving a newborn in daycare during the pandemic would put her child's health at risk. Eliana's reliance on her parents in contrast to Itzel being cut off from this support is an indication of the extent to which familial networks played a role in the ways women navigated decisions about returning to work. Even with family support, like many new parents, Eliana would have preferred to have more time with her newborn. Her return to work came with significant hardships. In multiple postpartum interviews, Eliana described feeling emotionally drained and often down, although she did not use the term depressed. She also struggled with breastfeeding and found it challenging to produce enough breastmilk with minimal breaks at work to pump. She finally decided to supplement her daughter's diet with formula, which she had been hesitant to do. Eliana's breastfeeding and emotional struggles align with research that shows the consequences of returning to work in a context of limited and often unpaid maternity leave in the United States (Kornfeind and Sipsma 2018; McCormack 2016).

Insecurities and Intimate Decisions

Throughout most of her pregnancy, Brisa had distanced herself from the baby's father, Juan Carlos. Worried that he was not ready for the responsibilities of parenthood, she thought it might be better to raise the child on her own. As the pregnancy progressed, Brisa became increasingly worried about how she would support the child. She had been living with a friend of *confianza*. In Spanish, a relationship of *confianza* entails trust and a sense of social obligation between people. Reflecting this deep connection was the fact that Brisa's friend did not charge her rent and shared whatever food she had so that Brisa would not go hungry. Despite their strong bond, Brisa grew worried that she would be exhausting her friend's goodwill after the baby arrived. When Juan Carlos reached out to her in the final months of pregnancy, Brisa accepted the support he offered. This included moving with Juan Carlos to his sister's house on the outskirts of the city. The couple married shortly after.

Prior to the birth, Juan Carlos encouraged Brisa to think about giving the baby formula so that they could put the baby in a daycare and both work. With two incomes, Brisa could begin to repay the money she borrowed almost three years prior. When Brisa returned to the hospital for several days with postpartum preeclampsia, she could not have the baby with her. The situation forced Juan Carlos to feed the baby formula. The baby refused the bottle, and when she did take it, she would vomit and become extremely fussy. When Brisa returned home from the hospital, Juan Carlos had a change of heart about their work plans. Instead of pushing her to return to work, he encouraged Brisa to stay home so that she could breastfeed, promising to support them and help repay her debts.

Although Brisa treasured having time with her baby, two factors continued to cause her significant anguish that she believed led her to have a diagnosis of postpartum depression. First, she continued to feel anxiety over her inability to repay her debts. Second, her new residence was in close proximity to a major Border Patrol facility. Brisa felt the presence of immigration enforcement everywhere she went. Even at night, Border Patrol helicopters swarming overhead frequently interrupted her sleep. As a result, she feared even going for walks outdoors with the baby. She said of seeing Border Patrol agents, "I feel like they know I am illegal."

As the baby approached her first birthday, Brisa received news that her mother's health was deteriorating. Brisa yearned to return to San Antonio to be with her mother. Juan Carlos also believed he could have opportunities for higher-paying work there. However, to return to San Antonio, the couple would have to cross an internal Border Patrol checkpoint where agents could potentially ask for identity documents.[2] For Juan Carlos, this was not a problem, given his status as a permanent resident. When Brisa first travelled to San Antonio from Mexico, she had done so using borrowed documents that she had since returned. Without valid documents, she had no easy way of crossing the checkpoint. When the couple heard that the checkpoint was temporarily closed, they quickly gathered whatever they could and took the opportunity to travel with an acquaintance to San Antonio.

In San Antonio, Brisa began to feel a sense of calmness she lacked in El Paso, primarily because she was away from the constant reminders of immigration enforcement. Many of the past tensions with her family members felt less intense as her family united in support of her mother. Further, Brisa was living with her mother, taking over many of the caretaker burdens from other family members. Yet, she was back in the same city as the woman who had lent her money. Even with some of her insecurities alleviated, Brisa had a constant fear over what measures this woman might take. She had been sending Brisa harassing messages with threats to take legal action. Brisa feared this could lead to the involvement of authorities and her deportation. Despite her continued anxiety, she was grateful for the time she was able to spend with her baby during the first year postpartum. Reflecting on the first year, she said, "To enjoy my baby—this is worth more than what we lack economically."

As the baby neared her first birthday, Brisa and her husband had devised a plan to improve their economic circumstances. They would both work, although Brisa would likely only be able to work part-time, needing to care for her mother and the baby. Brisa dreamt of finding a job that would allow her to bring her child but had come to terms with the idea that she would likely need to use a daycare. In making more money, first, the couple planned to save to pay back Brisa's loan. Then they would buy a small car to make it easier to take better jobs; at the time, Juan Carlos was travelling to work on a bicycle. Finally, they would save money to submit the paperwork to adjust Brisa's immigration status, which was a possibility following her marriage to a permanent resident.

Despite the numerous challenges she faced due to her economic and immigration-related insecurities, Brisa clearly enjoyed motherhood. She had a plan for making a more comfortable life for herself and her family. The insecurities she felt factored into the decisions she made about her intimate life, including her marriage to Juan Carlos. While Brisa felt that Juan Carlos had become more responsible and caring after the birth, she entered the marriage still uncertain of how their relationship would work out. Such pressures can lead precariously documented women into potentially abusive relationships (see Solis and Heckert 2021). Brisa's insecurities, exacerbated by the pandemic, significantly influenced her decision to marry in spite of her reservations.

Pandemic Benefits as a Safety Net

Sandra was in the second trimester of her third pregnancy when both her and her husband lost their jobs during early pandemic lockdowns. Given that only Sandra was able to receive unemployment, they struggled economically. Months following their layoffs, Sandra's husband found a new job. After the federal government expanded unemployment benefits during the pandemic, Sandra began to make more money than she did while employed. Jesus Cañas and colleagues (2022) show that Sandra was not alone in having a wage increase with unemployment. The federal supplements to unemployment of $600 per week meant that 62 percent of workers on unemployment in El Paso were receiving payments above their previous wages. Such figures fueled politicized arguments that the expanded unemployment benefits disincentivized returning to work. However, Sandra always intended to return to work. Her delayed return was a temporary response that enabled her to better care for her children. She felt relief that she was in this position to delay her return. In this sense, the pandemic enabled her to have a safety net that advocates of reproductive justice would argue should be ensured to all new parents to allow them time to bond with and care for an infant.

For Sandra, the expanded benefits during the pandemic offered protections that she otherwise would not have had. This allowed her to have income that essentially functioned similar to paid parental leave, which was a benefit she never had with past jobs. She contrasted this to her previous postpartum experiences, saying, "With my boys, I had to go back after the sixth week, and with her [the baby], I've actually been able to be home and enjoy her." Without the expanded unemployment benefits, Sandra would have felt forced to return to work while fearful of the risks to her daughter's health. Having previously worked in a childcare facility, she said, "I know how it is to work in a daycare. I'm not very happy about thinking that I would have to take my child to a daycare right now." As Itzel's experiences show, many women felt forced out of the workforce for similar reasons. Women's ability to receive unemployment was uneven and contingent upon the circumstances of their departure from their previous job. As Sandra's experiences show, support from unemployment could enable parents to better care for a newborn in the way they desired. Those without access to unemployment benefits, such as Itzel, faced profound struggles in deciding how to manage economic necessities while caring for a baby.

Childcare Challenges for Stay-at-Home Parents

While women who had already planned to stay at home with the baby often expressed little conflict over decisions about employment, they frequently described significantly more challenging caretaker burdens as a result of the pandemic. Alma gave birth to her seventh child in March 2021. Throughout most of her pregnancy, her five school-age children and toddler were home with her all day, every day. She described the challenges that virtual learning posed to her family:

> It was really hard at first because I had five in school and all of them were in different grade levels. I needed to make sure that my kids were listening. That they were paying attention. That they were doing their work. That if they had homework—even after the whole day being on

the computer they still had homework—I needed to make sure that I was doing all that. Plus my chores at home. Plus having something to eat. And I don't know, maybe just being at home makes them hungry all day, so they just wanted to be eating all day. I couldn't keep up with the housework, with the food, with their schoolwork. It was just really, really hard. That was a lot. I don't think I had said that out loud before.

While the labor of caretaking overwhelmed Alma, eventually she became numb to the pressure of always having too much to do. She explained, "Honestly, most of the time I feel like I don't have time to feel anything. Like my day is super-fast, and I don't know. I mean, obviously I'm tired, but I wake up. I never take my time to do something. How could I say it? Like it gives me like anxiety just to see someone taking their time. I just don't have time for that."

Just before the birth, Alma's five oldest children returned to school in person to complete the final months of the 2020–21 academic year. While this made the final weeks of her pregnancy as well as the newborn period easier to manage, it came with significant anxiety, as Alma feared one of the kids would bring COVID-19 home to the baby. As the pandemic continued, Alma's concern that the baby would contract COVID-19 only increased. Upon her children's return to school following summer vacation, it was becoming clear that the Delta variant was spreading rapidly among children. She explained how this affected her emotionally: "I was good until last night when they sent out a letter that one of the kids at my oldest daughter's school had COVID. We literally just started the school year two days ago, and we're back to kids getting COVID." Like many parents, Alma felt like she had no good options for her children, saying, "I want them to go to school and learn, but at the same time, I want them to stay home and be safe."

With the vaccine not yet available to children under twelve when the 2021–22 school year started, Alma had only been able to vaccinate her oldest child. Although she had some hesitancy in vaccinating her children,[3] she felt that the risks to her newborn outweighed the risks of vaccinating her children. Alma was well aware of how severe COVID-19 could be for more vulnerable age groups. In November 2020, her mother was hospitalized for two weeks with severe COVID-19. Alma at one point feared that her mother would not make it.

Alma's continued fear for her baby shows how the pandemic burdens persisted for parents with young children, even as the vaccine became available and pandemic restrictions loosened. Further, her caretaker overload, exacerbated by pandemic shutdowns, left her feeling completely drained on a day-to-day basis. This was a common pattern during the pandemic, especially for women who bore the brunt of additional caretaker work with school shutdowns (Laster Pirtle and Wright 2021). The fact that Alma said, "I don't think I had said that out loud before," after recounting her struggles during the pandemic, also reflects the emotional numbness that some people developed as a coping strategy during the height of the pandemic.

Disruptions to Family Unity for the Sake of Economic Security

Liliana had always planned to temporarily leave the workforce to be a stay-at-home mom while her children were young. When she became pregnant with her first child, she planned for her exit from her job as a nurse to take place one to two months before her due date in June 2020. Although the initial pandemic lockdowns caused her to move up her date of resignation, it did not create a dramatic disruption to her preexisting plan. However, her husband, Javi, being laid off shortly after the birth threw their family into economic turmoil. For several months, the couple had no income and a newborn to support. To pay their bills and buy groceries, they were borrowing thousands of dollars per month from family members.

Liliana and Javi soon realized that even if Javi found work locally, it would not pay enough to enable them to repay the money they had borrowed. They also knew that Javi could quickly find a job in the oil fields near Midland and Odessa, Texas. A typical starting salary in the oil fields for jobs without a college degree runs around $60,000 per year. In contrast, in El Paso, the median household income, a figure that encompasses households with multiple wage earners, is $51,325 (US Census 2021). However, taking a higher-paying job in the oil fields would require long hours and a six-hundred-mile round-trip commute from El Paso. Liliana and Javi decided that their best option for repaying their debt would be for Javi to take a job in the oil fields. A year and a half later, and the last time I spoke with Liliana, Javi was still gone for about a month at a time, returning for a week visit at most. During this period, Liliana became pregnant and gave birth to their second child in late summer of 2021.

In reflecting on their familial situation, Liliana expressed mixed emotions. She was grateful that Javi's job enabled her to stay at home with her babies, saying, "I'd rather stay with them at home and my husband supports me. He's working, trying to keep up with everything, so that I can stay with them." Yet, she also lamented at how their arrangement disrupted their familial unity, leaving her feeling isolated, lonely, and, at times, overwhelmed. Especially during the earlier stages of the pandemic, she was not yet comfortable having friends visit. Her parents had recently moved to Tennessee and her siblings could not cross the border from Juárez. Her loneliness led her to cry frequently. After the second birth, when Liliana had been fully vaccinated and was feeling more comfortable with social interaction, she had a close friend who would visit often. Further, her mother was able to come stay with her for a month. She feels like this emotional support kept her from falling into depression.

As Liliana became accustomed to long absences from her husband, she also felt like taking on everything on her own had helped her realize her own strength. Over two years into the pandemic, she reflected on what she had been through. "I've realized that I'm capable of a lot of stuff. That helped me with my self-esteem in a certain way, so that would be a positive thing that came out of all this mess," she said while laughing.

The pandemic precipitated the disruption to family unity experienced by Liliana. Her situation was not unique among the people we interviewed, as alluded to previously. Unable to find a decently paying job in El Paso, Lina's husband also took work in the oil fields shortly after the birth of their son. Anessa's husband took a short-term job working construction in Wyoming after the birth, primarily so the couple could save money to apply for Anessa's adjustment of status. During Jazmine's pregnancy, her husband took work that put him on the road for weeks at a time to enable the couple to pay their bills. This pattern shows that in an economically struggling region, where jobs are disproportionately concentrated in the low-wage sector, families often make significant sacrifices that involve a disruption to their family unit for the sake of just getting by. This puts enormous pressure on women who lacked the presence of a partner to share the labors of caretaking. It also limited men's abilities to be present in the lives of their children.

The Stress of Inflation

Even as the vaccine became available and COVID-19 therapies improved, women expressed trepidation over how returning to work could put their newborn's health at risk. Iris had left her job as a restaurant manager shortly before the birth of her third child. Not wanting to put the baby in a childcare facility, she had initially planned to stay at home for at least a year, as she had been able to do with her previous children. However, following the birth in the spring of 2022, rising prices meant that Iris's family was struggling to pay their bills. Feeling the pressures of inflation, Iris realized she would need to return to work earlier than planned and quickly found a new job that paid more than her previous position. Not wanting to expose her infant to COVID-19, rather than finding a childcare facility, her and her husband juggled their work schedules so that one of them could be home most days. For two days a week, Iris's mother would come stay with the baby. Again, it was the support of family that enabled Iris to feel comfortable about returning to work.

The pressure to return to work also created breastfeeding challenges in the midst of a formula shortage. Iris had exclusively breastfed her first two children until they were toddlers and hoped to avoid using formula with the new baby. The formula shortage made her even more adamant that she did not want to use any formula. Returning to work made feeding exclusively with breastmilk extremely difficult. Her work environment in a restaurant was not conducive for taking breaks to pump. Iris had prepared for this by storing as much breastmilk as she could in an extra freezer before her return to work. However, she was devastated when the freezer lost its power supply without anyone noticing, leading all her stored breastmilk to thaw and go bad.

The Bodily Effects of Powerlessness

Eight months postpartum, Lupe said, "I think my body is starting to break down the last couple of months. I think I'm a bit overwhelmed. I think I had a panic attack while at work on Thursday. . . . I'm trying my hardest [at work]. Like I know what I'm doing at my job. I'm good at my job, but it's just being there . . . especially with my son, 'cause he's so crazy, and it's just been a little overwhelming. I think my body is starting to really feel it."

Lupe's narrative, along with those of the other women presented here, reflect the significant emotional toll produced by the constraining circumstances of the pandemic during the postpartum period. As Lupe stated, these emotional struggles had bodily effects. For many women, the context of the border region played a significant role in how they experienced postpartum burdens. Women often felt powerless over the situations they faced, yet they found ways to persist. There has been significant attention to the ways such resiliency can have protective effects for individuals and communities. Attention to resiliency acknowledges the ways people exert agency, despite structural constraints. Yet, a focus on resilience comes with the risk of detracting attention away from the sociopolitical factors generating the crises people are facing (Barrios 2016). Additionally, the conditions that enabled resiliency were often related to various sources of privilege in women's lives. For example, Sandra's ability to receive unemployment enabled her to have more positive postpartum experiences. However, many women were not in a position that allowed them to have this source of income to ease their decisions about returning to work with an infant. Further, help from family members, particularly for childcare, was especially important for facilitating a return to work and easing economic hardships. Those with a precarious immigration status or cross-border families were less likely to have access to their family networks. Women's references to *impotencia* bring attention to the structural violence that serves as a backdrop to their everyday lives. The emotional struggles they experienced in relation to disempowering social structures should serve as a call to do better to ensure circumstances that enable people to thrive and raise families with dignity.

Impotencia and the Production of Reproductive Violence

The feelings of *impotencia* described by women were to a substantial degree produced by a lack of protections for parents during the postpartum period. Itzel, being a new employee at her company when she found out she was pregnant, had no protections under FMLA and felt forced to resign when limited to three weeks of leave following the birth. Eliana had leave, but it was unpaid, and she too felt forced to return to work before she was ready. To delay her return to work, she exhausted her savings, which stripped away her personal safety net. Iris initially planned to take more time off from work to care for her baby, but the economic pressures of inflation led her to return earlier than planned. The premature return to work for these women generated significant emotional distress from a postpartum overload, even for women who had various forms of social support that facilitated this return.

Some women found ways to spend more time with their infants, but this led to other sacrifices. Brisa continued to feel haunted by her inability to repay her debt. Liliana faced extended periods of separation from her husband so that he could pursue a job that would enable her to stay with the children. Sandra is one of the few women we interviewed who had the economic support that enabled her to stay home more easily with the baby. This did not come in the form of paid family leave, but rather, she was "lucky" enough to be fired rather than forced to resign. This detail allowed her to collect the extended pandemic-era unemployment benefits. In contrast, she felt forced back to work at six weeks postpartum following the births of her other children. Sandra's ability to have what mirrored paid parental leave provided tremendous relief and afforded her the opportunity to bond with her baby.

The struggles that women described postpartum existed before the pandemic and continue to exist now that the pandemic has subsided. The extent to which women feel this postpartum taxation is in large part a consequence of living in a country that has very few protections for parental leave and no federal policies to ensure paid parental leave. This lack of protection separates new parents from their infants before they are physically and emotionally ready. The pandemic made the stakes of decisions about returning to work far more complicated, as parents feared exposing their infants to COVID-19. Although the COVID-19 death rate for infants was relatively low when compared to other vulnerable groups, COVID-19 infection for infants came with a higher hospitalization rate, especially during the Omicron wave (Marks et al. 2022). Parents also feared the long-term implications of COVID-19 infection at such a young age. As the pandemic evolved, the availability of vaccines for the adult population led to a relaxation of preventive measures. This arguably put infants at an even greater risk by increasing their exposure while a vaccine for young children was not available until the summer of 2022. Infants under six months still cannot be vaccinated.

A lack of protective policies ultimately manifests as reproductive violence by disempowering new parents following the births of their children. This disempowerment may contribute to various forms of economic, social, emotional, and physical harm as well as pose limitations for parenting with dignity. Insufficient safety-net programs during the postpartum period contributed to disruptions to family units, women being overwhelmed with the tasks of caring for a newborn while feeling forced to return to work, persistent economic struggles, and overall feelings of emotional distress. The local context, which involved extended family separations from the border closure and additional stressors over immigration-related concerns, further exacerbated the hardships faced by some women.

While the pandemic undoubtedly made the postpartum period much more challenging for most women, some pandemic-era programs offer a glimpse into how safety-net programs can create more fulfilling postpartum experiences. The temporarily expanded Child Tax Credit helped Itzel make ends meet when her baby's father disappeared and she felt unable to return to work as quickly as her job demanded. Expanded unemployment benefits provided the safety net that Sandra needed to delay her return to work in order to care for her infant. These programs offer clear examples of what is possible at a national level in order to promote reproductive justice.

Conclusion

Imagining Reproductive Justice in the Borderlands

When I began drafting this conclusion, I was having trouble getting started, unable to escape the distracting sound of Border Patrol helicopters overhead. My home is mere miles from Sunland Park, New Mexico, an area where New Mexico, Texas, and Mexico meet. Sunland Park is just beyond the city bustle of El Paso and Juárez, making it one area where border crossers frequently attempt clandestine entry, even after public donations funded the extension of the border wall onto private land—terrain that is arguably unstable for structurally supporting the wall long-term. Border Patrol surveillance has always been heavy in the area, but it ramped up in response to the end of Title 42 on May 11, 2023, the date the COVID-19 public health emergency officially ended. Title 42 (also called the "Remain in Mexico" policy)[1] restricted the entry of asylum seekers under the pretext that migrants could introduce a communicable disease. With the inevitable end of Title 42, the media was reporting on an impending migrant crisis that quickly subsided. The state and federal governments responded through further militarizing the US-Mexico border.

When I drive from my home toward downtown El Paso along the César Chavez Border Highway, I often catch a distant glimpse of Border Patrol agents who are questioning a group of migrants. Often, they have turned themselves in to agents, as the beginning of an asylum claim. Occasionally, I witness Border Patrol vehicles chasing down clandestine border crossers. Such sightings are a part of daily life in El Paso. They remind me of the dream Brisa recounted of migrants crossing in dangerous circumstances, which she lamented, saying, "I dreamt they were my siblings." Many of us could learn something from Brisa's sense of kinship.

The Border Highway itself involves an elevated stretch that hovers over the border wall. Often as I drive, my cell phone begins to bounce

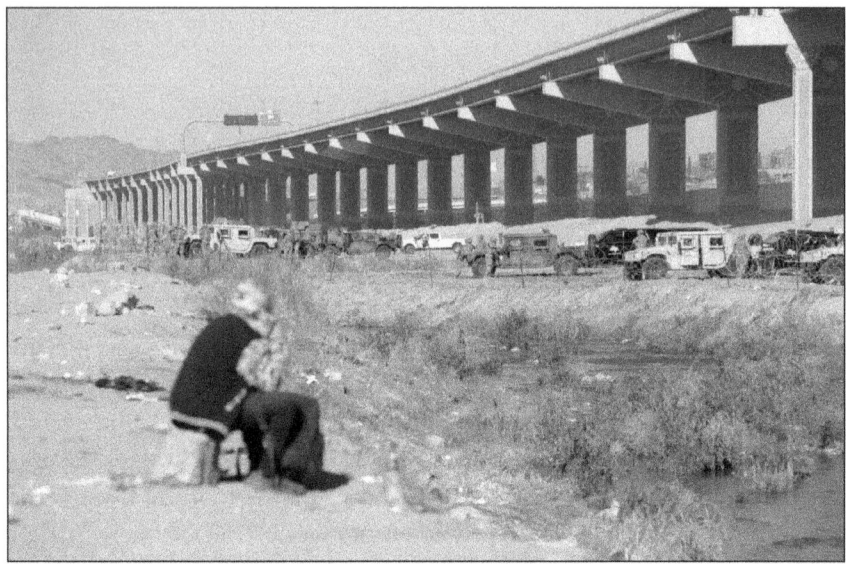

Figure C.1: The National Guard adds concertina wire on the US side of the border in December 2022
Credit: Corrie Boudreaux, *El Paso Matters*

off our neighbor's cell towers and I receive a "Welcome to Mexico" text message, even though I am still in the United States. Views from the highway provide glimpses into the increased military presence along the international boundary, which now includes an additional barrier of razor wire that separates the northern side of the Río Grande from a line of evenly spaced military tanks operated by the National Guard. As Title 42 came to an end, lines of asylum seekers formed at official and unofficial entry points into El Paso. Many of the migrants had young children with them. Some arrived at the border pregnant. In interviews with the press, people often repeated a variation of the same theme—they arrived at the border with a desire to raise their children and live their life with dignity and security.

What the media and politicians have framed as a border crisis involves a culmination of policies that have denied pathways of legal entry for those leaving untenable circumstances in their home countries, including violence and political and economic turmoil exacerbated by the pandemic. Title 42 blocked most pathways to seeking asylum. It relied on an agreement with Mexico that enabled the United States to return to Mexico asylum seekers from Mexico, Venezuela, Guatemala, Honduras, and El Salvador. Throughout its three-year lifespan, Title 42 was unevenly applied and constantly changing, allowing exceptions for people of some nationalities who the Mexican government would not accept and who could not be deported to their home countries.[2] Those from countries barred entry under Title 42 could attempt an unclear and confusing process to request an exemption, which could offer a pathway to receiving humanitarian parole. Often, migrants with limited options for legal entry have attempted clandestine crossing. Given the tight security of the border, a given individual may have various failed attempts at crossing, resulting in multiple encounters with authorities and inflating the statistics of attempted unauthorized entries. To be clear, there was a temporary significant increase in migrants arriving at the border in the lead-up to the end of Title 42. The inflation of the numbers of encounters with authorities, however, added fuel to politicized debates over immigration.[3] Further, these migrant flows quickly subsided.

Prior to the most recent claims of a border crisis, dehumanizing immigration policies already led migrants to increasingly dangerous and life-threatening methods of crossing the border and deportations into dangerous conditions (Slack 2019). When migrants and asylum seekers are stranded in Mexico, they may become subjected to extortion and state violence as well as institutional responses that offer inadequate protection. The March 27, 2023, fire in a migrant detention facility in Juárez that killed forty people who were awaiting the ability to claim asylum in the United States is one tragic example of the dangers migrants face in Mexico (Heyman and Slack 2023).

The current system for processing asylum seekers is insufficient for managing the number of people who may qualify for asylum. Those requesting asylum are temporarily held by immigration authorities. If an immigration official determines a person has a reasonable claim for asylum, they may be released on humanitarian parole while awaiting a court date that could be anywhere between six months and six years in the future. People granted humanitarian parole under the El Paso Border Patrol Sector are often left in the streets in downtown El Paso. Given that the Joe Biden administration attempted to end Title 42 prior to the end of the public health emergency only for legal decisions to allow the policy to remain in place, there were multiple instances when there was a significant spike in migrants at the border, as people hoped for a chance to request asylum after years of blocked options. During these spikes, on some days, Border Patrol released as many as ten thousand migrants into the streets. Migrants then needed to find shelter, food, and a way to continue their journey, rarely staying long-term in the border region. On two occasions—first in December 2022 and again in May 2023—El Paso Mayor Oscar Leeser declared a state of emergency to manage the number of people in need of food and shelter. This declaration enabled the city to use public properties to temporarily provide shelter to migrants. The State of Texas used both of these emergency declarations as a pretext to send the National Guard to the border.

Although Title 42 has officially ended, the Biden administration has now implemented policies that will have similar effects. Perhaps most significant is that asylum seekers traveling by land must apply and be denied asylum in a country that they have passed through in order to be eligible to apply for asylum in the United States. As past policies have demonstrated, efforts of deterrence force a shift in border crossing strategies and contribute to more dangerous clandestine crossings (Soto and Martínez 2018). Support for the most recent policies of deterrence hinges on the continued framing of a migrant crisis at the border.

This process of dehumanizing migrants seeps into entire communities subjected to the various forms of direct and indirect violence that characterize the region. The symbolic othering of the region as a zone characterized by foreign invasion is taken up as justification for continued violence within immigrant communities and in the border region. Telling was a public statement from Governor Greg Abbott following yet another mass shooting. On April 30, 2023, a gunman in Cleveland, Texas, murdered five of his neighbors, including a nine-year-old child. Abbott described the victims as "illegal immigrants." This statement was factually incorrect, as at least one victim was a US resident. More importantly, it reflects the denial of dignity to humans for political gain. It is a political strategy long used to justify the inhumanity of border policies.

Beyond the end of Title 42, the end of the public health emergency has other tangible effects. For over a year prior to the official end of the public health emergency, hospitalizations and deaths from COVID-19 had fallen dramatically from earlier points in the pandemic in large part because of vaccination, a high level of natural immunity at the population level, and less severe strains becoming the dominant variants of COVID-19. The reduced threat from the virus itself made the end of the emergency declaration inevitable. However, the world is still grappling with the aftershocks of the pandemic. The various traumas people went through during the pandemic may prove to have a range of lingering effects. The political and economic turmoil that the pandemic aggravated is driving displacement and migration. The pandemic put extreme pressure on health care workers, leading to widespread shortages of medical professionals that are likely to persist for years (ASPE 2022). More broadly, the pandemic intensified preexisting gender, racial, and socioeconomic inequities that are not easily remedied.

The official end of the public health emergency also brought an end to enhanced safety-net programs. Additional funding for nutrition programs such as SNAP means economically disadvantaged families have fewer food resources as they face increasing prices from inflation. It also brought an end to health care coverage for millions of people. A significant portion of the roughly two million Texans who gained coverage under Medicaid during the pandemic qualified due to pregnancy and maintained continuous coverage, at least on paper, through the duration of the public health emergency. An overwhelming majority of these individuals no longer qualify for Texas Medicaid, which has maintained strict eligibility criteria outside of the temporality of pregnancy. As women of reproductive age lose access to coverage under Medicaid, they also face growing restrictions on bodily autonomy. The *Dobbs v. Jackson* Supreme Court ruling has made abortion inaccessible in many parts of the United States, and Texas is among the states that has a total ban on the procedure. Telehealth services that may offer workarounds for ensuring access to medicated abortions in places where the procedure would otherwise be inaccessible are also at risk. Pending judicial decisions threaten a national ban on mifepristone, one of the drugs used in medicated abortions.

These events, characterized by long-standing patterns in the inhumane treatment of immigrants, gun violence, and insufficient access to health care, including abortion, are all matters of reproductive justice as they have a bearing on a person's abilities to exercise bodily autonomy and raise children with dignity and security. Limited access to health care, inhumane immigration policies, and exposure to an array of potentially harmful social and environmental circumstances in the context of diminishing social safety nets serve as sources of profound harm for women as they become pregnant, give birth, and care for their children. The concept of local biologies emphasizes that policies unfold in distinct ways in a given place and certain policies have contributed to a disproportionate burden of harm within the border region. My research took place during a particular period of time characterized by multiple sociopolitical and health crises. While current events and policies may evolve, there is a continued pattern of disproportionate potential for harm within the border region, especially for individuals in the most structurally vulnerable positions due to poverty, immigration concerns, and gender inequities. To ameliorate the harm caused by policies, it is imperative to reflect on what it would take to achieve a vision of reproductive justice.

Resisting Reproductive Violence

Envisioning reproductive justice in the El Paso region requires consideration of the contextual factors that have produced reproductive violence. Insufficient access to health care services, a high burden of poverty, border militarization, immigration policies, toxic environments, and the racialized othering of the region are among the factors that contribute to the disproportionate burden of ill health. Various manifestations of maternal harm are powerful indicators of this overall burden.

The reproductive justice movement considers how multiple social justice issues overlap in ways that manifest as reproductive oppression and maternal harm. As Patricia Zavella (2020) documents, during the Donald Trump administration, social justice movements felt a greater urgency to forge alliances to work toward overlapping goals and fight back against oppressive policies. In El Paso, such alliances have been especially important in mobilizing the community in response to the enactment of inhumane immigration policies. Perhaps most telling was the community's response to Trump's Zero Tolerance policy, which involved the deliberate separation of families seeking asylum at the US-Mexico border. Over a year and a half period, immigration authorities separated nearly four thousand children from their parents. Years later, nearly one thousand children still had not been reunited with their parents (DHS 2023). The community response in El Paso and elsewhere helped spur litigation that ended the policy of separating families, although there is evidence that border officials continued separating families following court orders. Community organizations in El Paso played an essential role in reuniting separated families. The strength of the community response in part came from the alliances across social justice movements and their shared recognition of the inhumanity of breaking apart families.

Community mobilization in response to a specific policy is but one means for resisting reproductive violence. Pragmatic solidarity is a useful term for envisioning pathways for achieving reproductive justice. The late medical anthropologist and physician Paul Farmer (2003) advocated for pragmatic solidarity, a term borrowed from liberation theology. It involves acting in a spirit of compassion to engage in actions to reduce social suffering. There are multiple levels and timeframes that go into practicing pragmatic solidarity. Given that many of the vulnerabilities that people face are direct consequences of social structures and inequitable policies, there is a need to make fundamental changes to how society operates. However, large-scale social changes are slow and uneven processes, while people have immediate needs. A pragmatic approach also requires attending to these immediate needs, even if it requires imperfect strategies.

Universal access to quality health care, regardless of a person's immigration status, is necessary to improve maternal and infant health by ensuring access to health resources before, during, and after pregnancy. The ACA served to fill in some important coverage gaps, but it fell short of creating universal coverage and maintained policies that exclude various immigrant populations from publicly funded programs. It is unlikely that an overhaul of the US health care system will occur in the near future, but there are smaller measures that could expand care for pregnant and postpartum people. Importantly, states now have the option to extend Medicaid for Pregnant Women to cover a person up to twelve months postpartum. As of August 2023, thirty-six states (including Washington, DC) had adopted this extension and ten others had plans to adopt it. In May 2023, the Texas legislature passed a law to extend coverage and the law was awaiting federal review to ensure it abides by federal guidelines. If the law goes into effect, it will be in large part the result of political advocacy and the work of reproductive justice groups that have been working for decades to expand postpartum coverage under Medicaid.

A continued limitation of Medicaid for Pregnant Women is that federal funds for the program maintain exclusions based on immigration status. There is an existing movement among health care workers to expand Medicaid to provide universal prenatal coverage (Fabi 2019). This expansion would help to reduce the inequities produced by the limited access to coverage granted under CHIP Perinatal. Such an expansion would be even more significant in states that do not currently offer coverage through the CHIP Perinatal option.

Women's overall positive experiences with midwives demonstrate the significance of having compassionate and structurally competent providers. However, there is a shortage of Certified Nurse Midwives (CNMs) in the region, which parallels a shortage of health care professionals in general. While there is a medical school in El Paso, it does not have a local CNM training program. Further, there are challenges in workforce retention in a medically underserved community. There are important regional endeavors aimed at building a health care workforce that reflects the demographics of the community, yet this will be a long-term project.

One possibility for providing women with more compassionate support during reproductive events is through expanded access to doulas. A doula is a birth support person who provides prenatal, labor, delivery, and postpartum assistance. Some doulas may also provide support for other reproductive health services, such as abortion. This type of support can help make a significant difference in people feeling empowered and respected during birth and when seeking other reproductive health services, especially among individuals with a more marginalized social position (Koumouitzes-Douvia and Carr 2006). Additionally, studies consistently show a reduction in adverse birth outcomes and fewer interventions in births where a doula is present (Gruber, Cupito, and Dobson 2013). Given that the training to become a doula is relatively quick and affordable compared to the cost and time necessary to become a midwife or physician, expanding access to doulas could possibly occur in a short timeframe. One challenge is that most insurance programs do not cover a doula and the cost of hiring one often makes this service inaccessible to lower-income individuals. Only one woman we interviewed hired a doula, although many women expressed a desire for this type of support. The inaccessibility of doulas for those with fewer economic resources makes it especially important to cover doulas through publicly funded programs. Oregon and Minnesota currently cover the cost of a doula through Medicaid. In March 2023, New York State passed legislation that allows coverage for doulas under Medicaid, after a pilot program showed this was a cost-effective strategy for improving birth outcomes. Additionally, some city and county programs cover doula services. Although Texas legislators have drafted legislation that would enable Medicaid to cover a doula, none of these proposals have passed a vote. El Paso currently has one private hospital that employs a limited number of doulas. While this is insufficient for making doulas widely available, it is illustrative of an additional way through which birth support could become more accessible within hospitals.

Beyond access to health services, structural circumstances within women's lives posed constraints and shaped their decisions about how to parent. These constraints were particularly salient around decisions about when to return to work in the midst of a public health crisis. Paid parental leave combined with enhanced access to social safety-net programs could help ensure people have dignified living conditions and the ability to care for and bond with an infant without having to make impossible decisions about returning to work. The pandemic-era expansions of safety-net programs offered additional protections for some people, showing what is possible and the differences that such policy shifts can offer people as they balance their economic concerns with a need to care for an infant. These temporary policies also revealed gaps in access to programs, and these gaps would need remedies to avoid further inequities. In particular, state policies that exclude immigrant populations serve as legal and bureaucratic violence. Any expansions to paid leave policies and other safety-net programs run the risk of deepening inequities if they continue to operate with a politics of exclusion. This brings up questions of how to support families within communities where the state has served as a source of reproductive oppression (see Rivkin-Fish 2013). Efforts of enhancing reproductive justice must include an approach that rejects exclusionary measures that would disproportionately harm not just immigrants but their families and communities as well.

Also significant to women in the border region are the stressors and traumas produced by immigration and border policies. As women's experiences showed, women perceive these policies as a significant source of harm for themselves and their babies. Advocates of humane immigration reform and border demilitarization recognize these are issues of reproductive justice, as current policies that separate families through deportation and deny people the ability to seek asylum prevent parents from having a sense of security in raising their children. More broadly, anti-immigrant sentiment casts the border as a racialized zone of foreignness. This symbolism has fueled the mistreatment and abuse of people in the region. Calls to demilitarize the border and enact immigration reform align with other racial justice priorities, including criminal justice reform and prison abolition, as the criminal justice system unfairly separates families and creates a disproportionate burden of trauma within communities of color.

The policy realms I have discussed are all areas where there is broad public support for reforms. Legislation to enact such reforms has in many cases reached a stalemate, in part due to political polarization. There is no easy solution to this political polarization and people's sense that their elected officials are failing to represent their needs and desires. This is especially true in Texas, where state-level policies have suppressed and disenfranchised voters.

Empowerment and social organizing have been key components of the reproductive justice movement and can help to counteract political disenfranchisement. Empowerment initiatives aim to provide people with education and tools that will enable them to recognize what has produced their structural vulnerability and allow them to see themselves as agents for changing these conditions. Through empowerment, communities can organize to resist and transform policies. Empowerment can mobilize multiple forms of individual, community, and political power (Zavella 2020). Mobilizing efforts have been central for shifting policies to protect women of color from forced and coerced sterilizations and challenging other sources of reproductive oppression (Gutiérrez and Fuentes 2009). Continued community organizing has the potential to shift policies and transform social structures over the long term.

Research also has power to drive policy shifts, yet there are issues in need of further investigation in order to better advocate for changes. Maternal health research focuses heavily on a limited set of variables, especially infant mortality, infant birth weight, maternal mortality, and severe maternal morbidity. With a limited scope of what is widely documented as indicators of maternal health, the more systematic, everyday forms of harm that women experience as a part of reproduction fail to register. When issues go under the radar, there is little attention to remedying these harms through policy shifts. As we have seen, the high rate of preeclampsia is one example of a widespread cause of maternal harm, as it contributes to adverse experiences. Yet, when adverse experiences do not escalate to an extreme outcome, they tend to receive little attention, in large part because of their lack of documentation in the places that matter.

There is also poor data on disparities in births covered under Medicaid for Pregnant Women in comparison to CHIP Perinatal and Emergency Medicaid. For example, the Pregnancy Risk Assessment Monitoring System (PRAMS), which is a Centers for Disease Control and Prevention (CDC) maternal health surveillance project, does an inadequate job of tracking outcomes for births covered under Emergency Medicaid or CHIP Perinatal. State health departments coordinate the collection of PRAMS data and have some discretion in what survey questions to include. In questions about health care coverage, most states lump all Medicaid programs together, prohibiting an analysis of how the differential coverage of these programs may be associated with disparate outcomes. An inability to make comparisons of these programs may hide the scope of some health issues related to a lack of comprehensive coverage by those who do not qualify for Medicaid for Pregnant Women due to their immigration status.

More systematic documentation of outcomes associated with births covered under CHIP Perinatal could support efforts to expand the range of services offered under this program. States have flexibility in deciding what to cover under CHIP Perinatal, and Texas is among the states with the most limited coverage. Expansion of the scope of CHIP Perinatal coverage could alleviate some of the inequities experienced by women covered under this program.

As broader transformations can be slow and uneven, there is a continued need for programs that meet people's immediate needs. In El

Paso, nonprofit community clinics serve as an important source of care for basic services. Several offer family planning services and prenatal care. One group of clinics also has a mobile unit and employs *promatoras* (community health workers) to provide outreach in some of the most marginalized sectors of the city. While these programs provide important services, with limited budgets, they are ultimately unable to meet all the complex health needs of structurally vulnerable populations with limited access to care.

* * *

In March 2022, Brisa reflected on her first year of motherhood. Numerous challenges marked that first year. Like many of the women whose stories I have been able to document, Brisa faced substantial hardship related to her economic precarity and immigration insecurities. The pandemic further exacerbated these adversities and, often, led her to feeling a sense of despair. Yet, even in this despair, Brisa navigated her circumstances as best she could in order to provide a better life for her daughter. She recounted joy over what it meant to become a mother: "When I see my baby, I feel it has been worth all the pain of everything that has happened. That's what I want to continue to have, for her to feel love and support. One year went so fast, and when I turned around to see her, I said, 'Good Lord, it's been a year.' And that's how the years pass. It's so beautiful for me. My daughter has returned life to me."

Brisa, and all parents, deserve better opportunities to have and raise children with dignity and security. Brisa should be able to live without fear that immigration policies will separate her from her daughter. Isabela should be able to send her children to school and other public places without anxiety that they will not return home after another mass shooting. Diana should not have to worry over being able to feed her family a healthy meal. Itzel should not have had to decide between economic stability and the health of her newborn during a public health catastrophe. Millions of children should be free of the burden created by unjust systems of incarceration and deportation that separate families. Everyone should have the security of being able to access basic health services. These are all matters of maternal health and reproductive justice.

ACKNOWLEDGMENTS

Countless people have supported the work that went into researching and writing this book. First and foremost, I would like to thank the women who shared a piece of their lives with me. This work would not have been possible without them. To protect their privacy, I cannot name them individually.

Many University of Texas at El Paso (UTEP) students assisted with all aspects of the research process. I am excited to see what each of them will accomplish in the future. Victoria de Anda, Isabela Solis, Jesus Aleman, Daniella Mata, James Milam, Cathy Román, Kimberly Anaya, Anamaria Solis, Rosario Olmos, Luis Torres, Star Chavez, Itzel Medina, Yamaris Cordero, Andrea Sandoval, Brianna Murillo, Donna Maldonado, Carolina Martinez, Alondra Arias, Dalia Hardy, Vianey Quaney, Sanjana Mada, and Nina Beltran provided valuable labor, analytical insights, and passion that helped keep this work going, especially during the COVID-19 pandemic. Cathy and Carolina in particular persisted during the most difficult phase of conducting research, over the phone and computer, as we maneuvered through the worst of the pandemic. I am honored that Victoria's artwork graces the cover of this book.

Ophra Leyser-Whalen, Naomi Fertman, Katie Serafine, Kristin Gosselink, and Adelle Monteblanco have been wonderful collaborators on various pieces of this work. At Texas Tech University Health Science Center–El Paso (TTUHSC–EP), Sireesha Reddy, Christina Bracamontes, Zuleika Curiel, Sheralyn Sanchez, and Madison Bencomo provided essential research support. Also (formerly) at TTUHSC–EP, Kristin Giroux and Nikki Skrinak shared valuable insights about providing compassionate care. Kristin also cared for me during my pregnancy and generously reviewed drafts of chapters 3 and 5.

Project Vida, Luna Tierra, Maternidad la Luz, Planned Parenthood of El Paso, and the Kelly Center for Hunger Relief are among the community organizations that have facilitated my work. Within these organizations I especially appreciate the support of Aída Ponce, Elena Carrillo, Ruth Kaufman, Warren Goodall, and Xochitl Rodriguez.

I was fortunate to have a wonderful writing group with colleagues in the Department of Sociology and Anthropology at UTEP. Cristina Morales, Angela Frederick, and Dean Chahim provided invaluable feedback, especially on chapter 3, which they helped save from being a chaotic mess. Other colleagues who have provided feedback and support at different stages include Jessica Lott, Saira Mehmood, Rachel Curtis, Regina Vadney, Nia Parson, Meghan Lowrey, Joe Heyman, Manny Campbell, Jeremy Slack, Heide Castañeda, Aurolyn Luykx, Selfa Chew, Sarah de los Santos Upton, Barbara Zimbalist, and Gina Núñez.

Chapter 2 draws heavily from an article previously published in *Ethos* and chapter 1 includes passages from a previously published article in *Human Organization*. Greg Downey and Nancy Romero-Daza as well as anonymous reviewers offered thorough and thoughtful feedback that improved those articles and helped me develop my ideas moving forward.

At NYU Press, Jennifer Hammer has been an enthusiastic and supportive editor from the beginning. Series editors Michele Rivkin-Fish, Paul Brodwin, and Susan Shaw as well as the anonymous reviewers provided valuable and constructive feedback that improved the final draft.

My work has been generously supported by the National Science Foundation Programs in Cultural Anthropology and Sociology through a Senior Researcher Grant (#1947551) and the Latino Center for Leadership Development through the Tower Center and Southern Methodist University. The UTEP Surpass, Meritus, and BUILDing Scholars Programs provided funding for students to work on this research. The BUILDing Scholars Programs is funded by the National Institute of General Medical Sciences of the National Institutes of Health under linked Award Numbers RL5GM118969, TL4GM118971, and UL1GM118970. The Faculty Development Research Leave program at UTEP enabled me to have valuable writing time. Thank you to Denis O'Hearn and Anadeli Bencomo for their support of this important program that can hopefully be expanded in the future.

While conducting the research for this book, I became a parent. Gabriel (Gabito) Saucedo Heckert has taught me about unconditional love.

Dario Saucedo has been a patient, kind, and loving husband in raising Gabito and in life. Our extended families in the United States and Bolivia have supported us in numerous ways both before and after we became parents. Gabito's grandparents, Sue and Paul Heckert and Ely and Dario Saucedo, are everything grandparents should be. Gabito is lucky that his Nana and Babo were so excited to meet him in the spring of 2020 that they took a pandemic road trip and drove twenty-four hours without stopping and repeated the feat several times while we remained in soft pandemic lockdown. His Abuela came to help care for him for six months when any other childcare scenario felt impossible. We are forever grateful for these acts of love from our family.

APPENDIX I

Integrating Cortisol Testing into Ethnographic Research

OVERVIEW

As a part of data collection from 2020 to 2022, we collected hair samples for cortisol testing from pregnant women recruited from a clinical context. These women also (1) participated in a survey that included sociodemographic questions and measures of emotional distress and (2) signed a HIPPA release to authorize access to medical records. The aim was to compare self-reported measures of emotional distress with a key biomarker of stress and stress-sensitive health variables.

Testing hair samples is one of many methods for assessing cortisol levels. Saliva, blood, urine, and fingernails are other bodily products that researchers have used for extracting cortisol. We chose to use hair samples, as it was the most feasible strategy within our overall research design. Cortisol levels in saliva, blood, and urine are ideal for measuring a person's current level of cortisol production. However, cortisol levels in these fluids are sensitive to a variety of factors, including the time of day, making it necessary to control for the time of day of the sample (Adam and Kumari 2009). Further, cortisol levels tend to increase during the second and third trimesters of pregnancy (Wosu et al. 2013). Given that we recruited patients during their prenatal appointments at various times of day and at different stages of pregnancy, it was not feasible to control for the range of factors needed to have good data from using saliva, blood, or urine.

Hair and fingernails store long-term data on cortisol (Russell et al. 2012). While providing hair samples may feel more invasive for many participants, hair does confer a distinct advantage when recruiting participants at different points in pregnancy. Since hair grows at a relatively consistent rate of 1.25 cm per month, it is possible to cut back hair samples to measure cortisol from hair that would have grown around the time of conception, in order to have a standardized baseline measure for all participants. While we had not seen this strategy used before based on our review of the literature, our initial analysis of the cortisol data suggests this strategy produced reliable data. An additional benefit of using hair is that samples can be stored at room temperature for a long period of time without risk of the cortisol degrading.

My own training as an anthropologist has been primarily in cultural anthropology, so I lacked the expertise and lab capacity to lead the analysis of cortisol data. Instead, Dr. Katherine Serafine, a neuroscientist at UTEP, oversaw the cortisol assays in her lab. I say this to emphasize that biocultural approaches do not have to be the sole territory of anthropologists with training across subfields. Rather, interdisciplinary collaboration is another means for collecting and analyzing biocultural data.

METHODOLOGICAL CHALLENGES DURING THE PANDEMIC

When we began data collection in September 2020, El Paso was on the verge of becoming one of the deadliest COVID-19 hotspots in the United States. Health facilities had extremely strict protocols in place. To be honest, I was surprised the medical school we were collaborating with permitted us to begin data collection. Even with permission to continue, I had my own hesitations. Primarily, I felt uneasy about potentially increasing the risks of exposure to COVID-19 for pregnant people and researchers. We decided to proceed given that all parties were required to wear masks and the clinic research staff were returning to in-person work regardless of whether we continued with the project or not. As a condition to collecting data, there could be no physical contact between research personnel and a participant. Further, researchers could not be in a room with participants for more than fifteen minutes. This timeframe was enough for the research assistant to explain the project, answer questions, go through informed consent, and explain how to complete the survey either over the phone or using a link to complete it online.

In order to conform to these guidelines, we developed a strategy for participants to take their own hair samples. To do this, we gave participants written instructions and sent a text message with a link to video instructions on taking the sample. Instructions included information on the necessary quantity of hair, the ideal location of the sample from the scalp, and the need for the sample to be taken from the root. Participants were asked to bring the hair sample to their next prenatal appointment. Even as pandemic restrictions eased, we continued with the same protocol to ensure consistency.

Beyond the context of the pandemic, there are other challenges in collecting hair samples. Some individuals may feel uncomfortable with providing a sample. Religious beliefs about exposing hair, the cultural associations between hair and beauty, and mistrust in how samples could be used are among the reasons a person might be hesitant to provide a hair sample (Wright et al. 2018). To be sensitive to these concerns, we decided to make providing a hair sample an optional part of participating in the overall study. In other words, a person could still complete the survey and participate in an interview while declining to provide a hair sample. Participants did receive an additional incentive for returning the hair sample.

In the end, 110 out of 176 participants provided a hair sample. Out of these samples, 61 were usable samples. Most of the unusable samples failed to have enough hair to extract a weight of hair sufficient for analysis. There were a small number of samples excluded for other reasons, such as appearing to come from the end of the hair strand, rather than from the root.

Clearly, self-sampling of hair did not result in the best samples. However, we believe that with some modifications, this strategy does offer some potential for future research. Self-sampling may help some people feel more comfortable with providing a hair sample, as it gives participants more control over the process. Our experience suggests some oversight is still necessary. This could include monitoring of the participant as they cut the sample, with the researcher providing feedback on whether the sample is of sufficient size and close enough to the root.

CORTISOL AND PREECLAMPSIA

A growing body of research suggests preeclampsia is stress sensitive and there is speculation that cortisol may play a role in the physiological pathway connecting experiences of stress to the development of preeclampsia (Vianna et al. 2011). However, data comparing cortisol to preeclampsia has been inconsistent. Some research shows higher cortisol levels among people who develop preeclampsia (Ho et al. 2007),

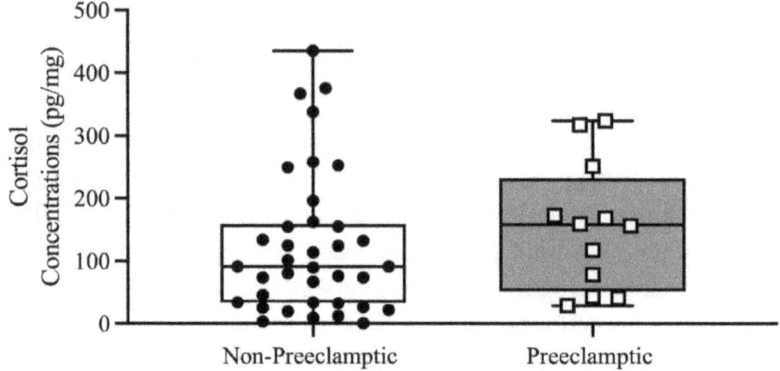

Figure A.1: Cortisol concentrations in preeclamptic vs. non-preeclamptic participants
Credit: Nina Beltran

while other studies show an unclear relationship (Sikkema et al. 2001). Our own data showed that women who developed preeclampsia had a higher median baseline cortisol level than those who did not develop preeclampsia (157.96 pg/mg compared to 91.41 pg/mg), although the difference was not statistically significant. Of the usable samples, only twelve were from women who developed preeclampsia. This small sample size limited our ability to show statistical significance (see figure A.1). It may also be the case that the timing of cortisol testing and the type of sample used are important for understanding how cortisol might play a role in preeclampsia. Joris Van Esch and colleagues (2020) found that steeper cortisol increases over the course of pregnancy, rather than a baseline measure alone, was predictive of early-onset preeclampsia. Nimesh Jayasuriya and colleagues (2019) found that the cortisol to cortisone (metabolized cortisol) ratio was significant. Pregnant people with a lower cortisol to cortisone ratio, meaning they were not metabolizing cortisol as efficiently, were more likely to develop preeclampsia. This cortisol metabolization may play a role in placental cortisol levels, and one study found that placental cortisol levels were higher in people with preeclampsia (Aufdenblatten et al. 2009).

As a whole, it seems that a single measure of cortisol, especially if it is a baseline reading, may not be a strong predictor of preeclampsia. However, cortisol fluctuations throughout pregnancy, best captured through multiple saliva, blood, or urine samples at multiple points in pregnancy, may produce better data. Metabolization of cortisol and placental cortisol levels may also be important variables to consider. It would likely require collaboration with medical researchers to collect this data. Beyond preeclampsia, we are in the process of analyzing the relationships between baseline cortisol levels and self-reports of emotional distress in relation to other maternal health variables and birth outcomes.

APPENDIX II

Participant Characteristics

TABLE A.1: Interview participant characteristics (2018–2019 study, n = 35)	
Type of prenatal coverage	
Medicaid for Pregnant Women	40%
Medicaid	2.9%
CHIP Perinatal	37.1%
Uninsured	11.4%
Private insurance	5.7%
Marketplace plan	2.9%
Immigration status	
US-born citizen	31.4%
Foreign-born US citizen	2.9%
Naturalized US citizen	8.6%
Permanent resident	25.7%
Unexpired temporary visa	14.3%
Undocumented	17.1%

TABLE A.2: Participant characteristics (2020–2022 study)

Type of prenatal coverage (Interview participants only, n = 60)	
Medicaid for Pregnant Women	71.7%
CHIP Perinatal	26.7%
Uninsured	1.7%
Immigration status (Interview participants only, n = 60)	
US-born citizen	68.3%
Naturalized US citizen	1.7%
Permanent resident	13.3%
Unexpired temporary visa	6.7%
Undocumented	10%
Prevalence of maternal health complications (Includes all survey participants, n = 176)	
Preeclampsia	24.9%
Gestational diabetes	24.7%
Dual diagnosis of preeclampsia and gestational diabetes	7.7%

APPENDIX III

Emotional Distress and Health Vulnerabilities

TABLE A.3: Social stressors, immigration concerns, and adverse birth outcomes

Pseudonym, Year of Interview	Immigration Concerns	Other Stressors	Notable Health Variables
Zahra, 2018	Permanent resident	Homeless while pregnant Economic insecurity Food insecurity	Preeclampsia Severe anemia
Aída, 2018	Permanent resident Previously undocumented Past deportation	None reported	Gestational diabetes Gestational hypertension
Margot, 2018	Undocumented	Son with special needs Economic insecurity	Gestational diabetes High blood pressure
Martha, 2018	Permanent resident Previously undocumented	History of abuse (gained residency under VAWA*)	Depression Gestational diabetes High blood pressure Anemia
Tamara, 2018	US-born citizen	Brother murdered in Mexico History of abuse	Preterm birth Near infant mortality
Rita, 2018	Undocumented, adjusting status under VAWA	History of abuse Economic insecurity	Gestational diabetes
Sofi, 2018	Undocumented, adjusting status under VAWA	History of abuse Economic insecurity	First two pregnancies: Low birth weight
Marla, 2019	US-born citizen Husband deported	Economic insecurity Son has behavioral issues tied to separation from father	First pregnancy: Preeclampsia Preterm birth Low birth weight Second pregnancy: Gestational hypertension Infant respiratory distress

TABLE A.3 (cont.)

Pseudonym, Year of Interview	Immigration Concerns	Other Stressors	Notable Health Variables
Julia, 2019	Naturalized US citizen Previously undocumented Undocumented family members	Relationship problems	Gestational diabetes Preterm birth
Aurelia, 2019	US-born citizen Mother previously undocumented and deported multiple times As child, held in detention with mother	Caring for younger siblings who live with abusive father	Low birth weight
Sandra, 2021	DACA recipient Husband undocumented	Lost job during pandemic Childcare issues during pandemic	Preeclampsia Type 2 diabetes
Lupe, 2021	US-born citizen	No support from child's father	Preeclampsia Postpartum hemorrhage Returned to ER for postpartum preeclampsia Postpartum depression
Salma, 2021	US-born citizen Mother and sister undocumented	History of abuse Traumatic childhood Food insecurity throughout childhood	Type 2 diabetes
Janeth, 2021	US-born citizen Family members seeking asylum were deported In-laws in process of adjusting status	Children with preexisting conditions Extreme pandemic-related anxiety Husband lost job during pandemic Economic insecurity	Low birth weight Gestational diabetes Preeclampsia Severe depression during pregnancy and postpartum with suicidal thoughts
Alma, 2021	US-born citizen	Childcare challenges during pandemic Economic insecurity	Preterm birth First trimester COVID-19 hospitalization Placenta accreta
Eliana, 2021	US-born citizen	Complicated relationship with baby's father Economic insecurity Fears of contracting COVID-19 through high-risk job	Gestational diabetes

TABLE A.3 *(cont.)*

Pseudonym, Year of Interview	Immigration Concerns	Other Stressors	Notable Health Variables
Brisa, 2021	Undocumented	Economic insecurity	Preeclampsia
		Fears of returning to work during pandemic	Postpartum hemorrhage
			Manual placenta removal
Itzel, 2021	Born in US, USCIS denied her passport application due to circumstances of birth	Economic insecurity	Gestational diabetes
		Food insecurity	
		Lack of support from baby's father	
		Separation from family with border closure	
Isabela, 2021	US-born citizen Immigration concerns for family members	Developed anxiety following the mass shooting	Symptoms of long-COVID
			Low blood pressure
		Challenges getting mental health support during pandemic	Depression
			Anxiety
			Anemia
Lina, 2021	US-born citizen, grew up in Juárez	Abuse in household growing up	Low birth weight
			Preeclampsia
		Interpersonal challenges with family	Fetal hydrocephaly
Liliana, 2021	Permanent Resident via marriage	Loss of income during pandemic	Gestational diabetes
	Father has history of deportation	Husband took out-of-town job to repay loans	
Juliana, 2021	US-born citizen	High level of fear from the pandemic	Postpartum hemorrhage
	Sister undocumented and deported		Hospitalized 3 times during pregnancy due to dehydration from severe morning sickness
Anessa, 2021	Adjusting status via marriage to US citizen	Challenges living with in-laws	COVID-19 during delivery
		Separation from family members during border closure	Mastitis
			Postpartum depression
		Husband took job out-of-town to alleviate economic concerns	
Talia, 2021	US-born citizen	Boyfriend COVID-19 positive at time of birth and unable to be present until weeks later	Preeclampsia
			Anemia
			Vitamin B12 deficiency
		Boyfriend in military and deployed shortly after the birth	

* VAWA (the Violence Against Women Act) allows undocumented immigrants to self-petition for US residency if they have been the victim of intimate partner violence and were married to a US citizen or permanent resident.

NOTES

INTRODUCTION

1 Throughout the book, I alternate between using pregnant person and pregnant woman. The term pregnant person aims for greater inclusivity, acknowledging that a person with a diverse gender identity who does not identify as a woman may have a uterus and the capacity to become pregnant. However, it is also important to push back against a legacy and practices that have made women invisible in medicine. Using the term woman is an effort to demand the visibility of the female body and gendered experiences. There are linguistic challenges in maintaining inclusivity while also demanding attention to the gender inequities in medicine that harm women. My response has been to use gender neutral language when speaking broadly about the processes of reproduction. When I move into my own data, in which every person I interviewed identified as a cisgender woman, I tend to shift into gendered language, in part to account for the gendered dimensions of these individuals' experiences. I realize this is an imperfect strategy for dealing with the linguistic limitations for describing highly gendered experiences.

2 States have the option to waive the five-year waiting period for coverage under Medicaid for Pregnant Women. However, Texas does not offer this waiver. Further, the bureaucratic measures used to establish the length-of-residency requirement in Texas may serve to exclude immigrants who have legal residency beyond five years. To meet the length-of-residency requirement, a person must have initiated the process to become a naturalized citizen or have earned forty quarters of Social Security credits between themselves and a spouse (Texas DSHS, n.d.). If a person has not naturalized, is unmarried, has a spouse who has been out of the workforce, or has not been in the workforce for the full duration of their legal residency, which is often the case for women taking care of young children, they may still be excluded from Medicaid for Pregnant Women.

3 Five states and the District of Columbia use state and local funds to expand coverage for some immigrant populations. For example, Colorado uses state funds to cover Marketplace premium costs to low-income individuals regardless of immigration status and California extends Medicaid to adults ages nineteen to twenty-six and over the age of fifty regardless of immigration status (KFF 2023). Some pregnant people may gain coverage through such mechanisms.

4 Jeremy Barofsky and colleagues (2020) conducted a county-level analysis and found that following the October 2018 announcement of planned changes to the

likely public charge rule, for every 1 percent increase in the immigrant population of a county, there was a 0.1 percent decline in the use of child Medicaid programs. They did not analyze data specific to CHIP Perinatal.

5   This practice extends beyond the border region. For example, a Miami hospital advertises services to affluent parents throughout Latin America, offering birth packages, temporary accommodation, and information on the legal mechanisms for travelling to the United States for the birth (see Have My Baby in Miami 2021).

6   Working book manuscript.

7   This figure should be viewed cautiously. US citizens and permanent residents living in Juárez were able to cross the border to be vaccinated in El Paso. While the border remained closed, individuals with other types of visas could still cross for essential purposes, including work, school, and seeking health services. Border Patrol agents have significant discretion in admitting individuals under these criteria, so a vaccination appointment could be used as grounds for admission, depending on the agent. As a part of mass vaccination efforts, neither the city nor county requested proof of residency in Texas in an attempt to make the vaccine more easily accessible to anyone who wanted it. This measure also made it impossible to track how many vaccines were administered to people who reside primarily in Juárez, potentially skewing estimates of the total vaccination rate in El Paso.

8   The CARES Act was an economic stimulus bill aimed at alleviating the economic repercussions of the COVID-19 pandemic. It included economic stimulus payments and temporarily expanded unemployment benefits. Undocumented immigrants were excluded from receiving stimulus checks.

1. LEGISLATING MATERNAL HARM

Sections in this chapter were previously published in "The Bureaucratic Violence of the Health Care System for Pregnant Immigrants on the United States-Mexico Border." *Human Organization* 79, no. 1 (2020): 33–42.

1   The Women, Infants, and Children (WIC) program uses federal funding to support state programs that provide nutrition supplements and education to low-income pregnant women and families with children under the age of five. In Texas, recipients receive benefits based on their number of qualifying children. The mother receives additional benefits for herself if she is pregnant or postpartum. These benefits include access to a lactation consultant.

2   Significant changes to Medicaid during the 1980s resulted in expanded coverage during pregnancy and did not initially involve exclusions based on immigration status. In 1986, federal legislation provided states with the option of covering all pregnant people with an income below the federal poverty level (FPL). The following year, the income cutoff increased to 185 percent of the FPL. By 1990, rather than states having the option to cover pregnant people under Medicaid, they were required to cover anyone below 133 percent of the FPL (Ellwood and Kenney 1995). It was not until the Personal Responsibility and Work Opportunity Act of 1996 that immigration status was used as a grounds for exclusion from Medicaid

programs, creating a distinction between deserving and undeserving immigrants (Viladrich 2012). Since 1996, other than an exception for Emergency Medicaid, federal policy prevents the use of federal Medicaid funds to provide healthcare coverage for unauthorized immigrants, although New York, Massachusetts, and New Jersey use state funding to extend Medicaid for Pregnant Women to those who would otherwise be excluded based on immigration status. Under the Affordable Care Act (ACA), Texas opted out of Medicaid expansion for the general population but did expand Medicaid for Pregnant Women to cover individuals up to 198 percent of the FPL for the pregnancy and sixty days postpartum.

3   Additionally, federal funds cannot be used for postpartum care, with the exception of covering postpartum visits if they are included in a payment bundle with the prenatal care and delivery. Nine states use state funding to provide more comprehensive services during pregnancy and the postpartum period under CHIP Perinatal, making it comparable to what is covered under Medicaid.

4   There is evidence that expanding prenatal care under CHIP Perinatal is cost effective. For example, Maria Rodriguez and colleagues (2020) found that it costs an average of $380 more per birth to provide coverage under CHIP Perinatal as opposed to Emergency Medicaid. However, given the associated reduction in infant mortality, infant morbidity, and NICU (neonatal intensive care unit) stays, the overall cost to the health care system is lower. Yet, such evidence is not what facilitated the passage of CHIP Perinatal in Texas.

5   Title X clinics provide reproductive health services and contraception using federal grant money allocated to states. Some Title X clinics are able to provide limited prenatal care, most often through CNMs or nurse practitioners, although more advanced screenings and tests are usually not available. The reliance on Title X clinics for the provision of care reveals contradictions in Medicaid polices. While federal funding for Medicaid involves exclusions based on immigration status, federal funding to Title X clinics subsidizes Medicaid programs by providing care to those excluded from Medicaid (Boehm 2005).

6   Recipients of HTW are subjected to an annual review process and may lose coverage if their family income goes above 202.4 percent of the FPL.

7   "Intended miscarriage" is not a medical term. Rather, it reflects a particular political agenda aimed at denying people coverage under Medicaid if they had an abortion.

2. IMMIGRATION POLICY AND EMBODIED VULNERABILITIES

An earlier version of this chapter was published as "Embodied Pathways of Emotional Distress and Birth Complications among Immigrant Women on the US-Mexico Border." *Ethos* 48, no. 4 (2021): 438–58.

1   Anahí, whom we interviewed in 2018, delivered at a private hospital, in contrast to the participants in our 2020–22 study who planned to birth at the county safety-net hospital. This is an important distinction given varying hospital policies and providers contribute to significant variations in the management of labor

and delivery, with C-section rates reflecting one dimension of these differences. I further discuss this issue in chapter 5.

2   In the month following our interview, wait times to cross the border increased dramatically, and reports of six-hour wait times were common. The wait times were in part a consequence of the Trump administration reassigning Border Patrol officials away from ports of entry. Instead, Border Patrol agents began patrolling the international boundary in an effort to stop asylum seekers from stepping foot onto US soil. Seemingly, the goal was to prevent asylum seekers from arriving at ports-of-entry, which are on US soil. Once a person is on US soil, they have a legal right to request asylum. If they are never able to cross the line onto US soil, Border Patrol agents do not have to consider these claims.

3   Although the War on Drugs dates to the Richard Nixon era, violence in Mexico did not begin to spike until the mid-2000s (Shirk 2010). This is in part because prior to this period, drug trafficking routes from South America operated primarily by sea and air. As the War on Drugs began to increase the risks of trafficking by air and sea, cartel routes shifted to land, running from South America through Central America and Mexico. By 2007, an estimated 90 percent of all cocaine trafficked into the United States came through Mexico. During this same period, it also became increasingly easy for Mexican cartels to obtain assault rifles from the United States; the 2004 lift on the assault rifle ban in the United States can partially explain the rise in homicide rates in Mexico (Chicoine 2016).

The Mérida Initiative, a 2008 agreement between the United States and Mexico aimed at reducing drug trafficking, has been criticized for further fueling cartel violence. This initiative pumped hundreds of millions of dollars annually into the Mexican military with the goal of combating cartels. The Mérida Initiative followed Mexican president Felipe Calderón's declaration of war against the cartels, thus the Mexican government welcomed this initiative at the time. However, rather than weakening the cartels, the use of warfare tactics by the police and military led to a dramatic increase in cartel violence, widespread corruption within law enforcement, and strengthening of the cartels (Rosen and Zepeda 2016; Vogt 2017).

4   This account is supported by a well-documented pattern that both acute and chronic stress are associated with preterm birth (Dunkel Schetter and Glynn 2011).

3. THE LOCAL BIOLOGY OF PREECLAMPSIA

1   Eclampsia was one of the first medical conditions documented in writing, with accounts originating in India, China, Africa, and Europe dated as far back as 3000 BC. Many cultures throughout history have attributed eclamptic seizures to spirit possession. It is perhaps the high death rate of untreated eclampsia that has made the condition the subject of intense social and medical speculation throughout history (Robillard et al. 2017).

2 The abnormal placentation involved in preeclampsia increases the risk of hemorrhage for both vaginal and cesarean deliveries. Additionally, magnesium sulfate, which is the primary treatment for managing the hypertension resulting from preeclampsia, increases the risk of hemorrhage.
3 This figure includes one case of eclampsia.
4 A common strategy for estimating prevalence rates of preeclampsia involves a review of electronic medical records. A larger scale review of medical records beyond what we conducted for our research participants would have been an extremely laborious process that was beyond the capacity of data collection that we could complete for our study.
5 Among Mexican-origin women within the Gong et al. (2012) study, there may have been significant differences in relation to immigration status, socioeconomic status, and geographic residence throughout the life course, however, they lacked sufficient data to analyze these variables. Further, the higher prevalence rate among Mexican-origin women does not suggest there is anything about Mexican nationality that generates this risk; rather, it points to a need to consider what might constitute shared social and environmental risks, including experiences of racism and xenophobia (Fasanya et al. 2021).
6 We also found a high prevalence rate of gestational diabetes within our sample. Of 176 participants, 24.7 percent had a diagnosis of gestational diabetes, compared to a national prevalence rate of 8.3 percent in 2021 (CDC 2023). Within our sample, 7.7 percent of women had a dual diagnosis of gestational diabetes and preeclampsia. Slightly less than one-third (31.7 percent) of women who developed preeclampsia also had gestational diabetes. In this chapter, I decided to focus on preeclampsia primarily because there has been very little ethnographic investigation of this condition, despite the fact that it is a leading cause of maternal mortality and morbidity.
7 A maquiladora is a manufacturing plant where raw goods can be imported into Mexico's free trade zone for assembly. Final products are exported tax-free.
8 Political moves have at times led to increased wait times, resulting in an even greater burden of air pollution. For example, in April 2022, Governor Greg Abbott announced plans to implement additional inspections of trucks entering the United States, as a part of his protest over what he described as President Joe Biden's failure to secure the border. Abbott was later forced to halt these inspections when trucks experienced day-long delays in crossing that led to a significant disruption in commerce.
9 The release of cortisol in particular weakens anti-inflammatory responses that lead to increased oxidative stress and endothelial dysfunction—important in the pathways involved in preeclampsia.
10 There is some evidence that due to the similarities in the pathological indicators of COVID-19 and preeclampsia, perhaps there were some mistaken diagnoses of preeclampsia, especially early in the pandemic when researchers were still trying to understand COVID-19 (Mendoza et al. 2020).

11 For example, following COVID-19 infection in early pregnancy, Alma was diagnosed with placenta accreta. Placenta accreta occurs when the placenta grows too deeply into the uterine wall. Because the placenta cannot easily detach, the condition can easily lead to life-threatening hemorrhaging. Alma received the recommended protocol of having a C-section and total hysterectomy to avoid complications.

12 In our experience, it is extremely difficult to collect good data on COVID-19 infection during pregnancy. As such, there may be an even stronger relationship between COVID-19 and the development of preeclampsia than what the literature already shows. In collecting data from electronic medical records, we noted if the records indicated COVID-19 infection during pregnancy. In comparing interview data to medical record data, we found many self-reports of COVID-19 infection during pregnancy that were not reported in medical records. It seems the absence from medical records was particularly strong if the woman reported COVID-19 infection early in the pregnancy prior to initiating prenatal care. Within our survey data, we did ask about COVID-19 infection. Given that many women completed the survey early in their pregnancies, our survey data is a poor indicator of COVID-19 infection throughout the duration of pregnancy.

13 However, there is mixed evidence on whether or not induction for diabetes is always medically necessary, as variables such as glycemic control may play a significant role in birth outcomes (Dekker 2019). A tendency to overmedicalize birth may contribute to the routine practice of inducing labor for a pregnant person with diabetes, as induction gives providers more control over the birth. The fact that induction rates in the United States have tripled over the past three decades (Simpson 2022) offers further evidence of the increasing tendency for physicians to use the technologies at their disposal to control the natural process of birth. However, there are additional factors to consider. Throughout the Unites States, labor and delivery wards have been closing in rural and isolated areas. This pattern limits options for pregnant people and can contribute to excessively long travel times during labor. In such circumstances, induction can offer a pregnant person some power and security in accessing care (Pearson et al. 2018).

14 African American women, women over the age of forty, and women with a body mass index (BMI) greater than thirty also have increased risk for postpartum preeclampsia (Bigelow et al. 2014).

15 Additionally, diagnostic criteria that relies on blood pressure and proteinuria may be inadequate for detecting the condition. While hypertension is the most common manifestation of preeclampsia, it is not always present and other signs of organ damage may be progressing in absence of a timely diagnosis (Von Dadelszen and Magee 2014).

4. CONJUGATED HARM AND PREGNANCY DURING THE PANDEMIC

1 Bourgois also argues that conjugated oppression has been essential for the expansion of capitalism. He is particularly concerned with how racial and ethnic

ideologies perpetuate class hierarchies, with the resulting oppression operating to benefit capitalist systems.
2   This is not to imply border traffic only flows north. Border crossing is bidirectional, but there is better record keeping of northbound flows.

5. FINDING COMPASSIONATE CARE

1   In using the term baby, I am relying on Brisa's words. My aim is to show sensitivity toward how Brisa felt about her pregnancy and miscarriage. I do not intend for this to be a statement suggesting that a nonviable fetus is a baby.
2   Five states also license Certified Midwives (CMs). CMs have a graduate-level midwifery education that does not include nursing, distinguishing it from the CNM licensure. Despite this difference, CNMs and CMs have to pass the same board exams and can both practice in hospital settings.
3   In 1976, the Midwifery Center of El Paso opened the first midwifery school in the city. After closure of the Midwifery Center, in 1987, Maternidad la Luz opened a midwifery school that is self-described as the "Harvard of Midwifery School" (Anchondo-Rivera 2016).
4   The longest-serving group of FQHCs in El Paso is Centro de Salud Familiar La Fe. In 1969, a group of Chicano/a activists founded the center. Despite the first clinic's association with the Catholic Church, the center always had a focus on reproductive health services. Leaders even renamed the clinic, which had initially been Father Rahm Clinic, to prevent residents from assuming that they could not access birth control there because of its ties to the Catholic Church (Murillo 2016).
5   Over the last several decades, there have been increased efforts to train healthcare workers in cultural and structural competency as a way to better serve vulnerable populations. There is significant variation in structural and cultural competency curriculums within different health professions and unevenness in how providers interpret and apply the training in clinical contexts (Kleinman and Benson 2006; Metzl and Roberts 2014).
6   Border Patrol agents may be able to see if there is an active warrant for an individual. While a warrant cannot be issued for unpaid medical bills, debt collectors may attempt to take a person to debtor's court. If a person fails to appear in court, a judge could issue a warrant. However, Texas public hospitals cannot send a bill to collections to begin with if the patient has not first received information on discount programs and payment plan options. According to Celeste, the hospital did not offer her these options.
7   This scarcity is increasingly a problem in rural and geographically isolated areas that have experienced closures of entire maternity wards in an effort to save hospitals money.

6. NAVIGATING *IMPOTENCIA* DURING THE POSTPARTUM PERIOD

1   The American Rescue Plan increased the 2021 Child Tax Credit from $2,000 per child to $3,000 per child over the age of six and $3,600 per child under the age

of six. Instead of having to wait for payment of the tax credit until after filing tax returns, the federal government issued the credit through monthly payments. The increased tax credit expired in 2022.
2 Border Patrol operates thirty-three permanent checkpoints located on major highways between twenty-five and seventy-five miles of the US-Mexico border. Legally, US citizens do not need to provide proof of citizenship to pass through the checkpoints, however, the American Civil Liberties Union (ACLU) has documented what appears to be a pattern of racial profiling where people "suspected" of being undocumented are routinely asked for documentation. This practice has led to at least three hundred wrongful arrests of US citizens. As such, the ACLU has engaged in legal measures that argues that the checkpoints are unconstitutional and a violation of Fourth Amendment rights (ACLU 2021).
3 Alma's concern reflects a broader trend. Latino/a and Black parents may be especially hesitant to vaccinate young children due to mistrust in health authorities (Alfieri et al. 2021).

CONCLUSION

1 Title 42 originally went into effect in March 2020 during the Donald Trump administration. The Joe Biden administration delayed ending Title 42, despite the lack of any credible public health evidence that it helped control the spread of COVID-19 in the United States. When the Biden administration first attempted an end to Title 42, subsequent court rulings stalled the end of the policy.
2 Critics of Title 42 have pointed to how race has factored into exceptions under the program, as an unlimited number of Ukrainians could request asylum. In contrast, political turmoil has led over 25 percent of the Venezuelan population to leave the country, yet when the Biden administration amended Title 42 to accept some Venezuelans, the amendment included quotas and mechanisms to deter those seeking protection.
3 Prior to the end of Title 42 in May 2023, it appeared that the program would end in December 2022. However, the Supreme Court ordered that restrictions could remain in place. The end of the public health emergency made it unjustifiable to continue to implement Title 42 under the pretext of public health. Each time that it appeared that Title 42 would end, there was an influx of asylum seekers at the border in anticipation of possible new options for legally entering and requesting asylum. On each occasion, the state and federal governments responded through increased border militarization.

BIBLIOGRAPHY

Abrego, Leisy, and Sarah Lakhani. 2015. "Incomplete Inclusion: Legal Violence and Immigrants in Liminal Legal Statuses." *Law and Policy* 37 (4): 265–93.

Abrego, Leisy, and Cecilia Menjívar. 2011. "Immigrant Latina Mothers as Targets of Legal Violence." *International Journal of Sociology of the Family* 37 (1): 9–26.

Abrego, Leisy, and Leah Schmalzbauer. 2018. "Illegality, Motherhood, and Place: Undocumented Latinas Making Meaning and Negotiating Daily Life." *Women's Studies International Forum* 67:10–17.

Adam, Emma, and Meena Kumari. 2009. "Assessing Salivary Cortisol in Large-Scale, Epidemiological Research." *Psychoneuroendocrinology* 34 (10): 1423–36.

Alexander, Barbara. 2007. "Prenatal Influences and Endothelial Dysfunction: A Link between Reduced Placental Perfusion and Preeclampsia." 49 (4): 775–6.

Alfieri, Nina, Jennifer Kusma, Nia Heard-Garris, Matthew Davis, Emily Golbeck, Leonardo Barrera, and Michelle Macy. 2021. "Parental COVID-19 Vaccine Hesitancy for Children: Vulnerability in an Urban Hotspot." *BMC Public Health* 21:1–9.

Allen, Steve, Eric Barkley, Denise Rasmussen, Neil Sandburg, and Harry Freedman. 2022. "Hospitalization Risk for COVID-19 Positive Infants Six Times Higher than Other Kids Under 5." *Epic Research*, April 29, 2022. https://epicresearch.org.

Alvord, Daniel, Cecilia Menjívar, and Andrea Gómez Cervantes. 2018. "The Legal Violence in the 2017 Executive Orders: The Expansion of Immigrant Criminalization in Kansas." *Social Currents* 5 (5): 411–20.

American Civil Liberties Union (ACLU). 2021. "Federal Court Allows ACLU Case Challenging Border Patrol's Use of Checkpoints to Proceed." ACLU, April 9, 2021. www.aclu.org.

American College of Obstetrics and Gynecology (ACOG). 2020. "Gestational Hypertension and Preeclampsia: ACOG Practice Bulletin." *Obstetrics and Gynecology* 135 (6): e237–60.

American Immigration Council. 2022. *Rising Border Encounters in 2021: An Overview and Analysis*. American Immigration Council, March 4, 2022. www.americanimmigrationcouncil.org.

American Lung Association. 2021. *State of the Air*. Chicago: American Lung Assosiation.

Anchondo-Rivera, Anessa. 2016. "*Esta con la Partera:* A Qualitative Feminist Perspective of Women's Birthing Experiences in El Paso, Texas." MA, Department of Sociology and Anthropology, University of Texas at El Paso.

Andaya, Elise. 2018. "Stratification through Medicaid: Public Prenatal Care in New York City." In *Unequal Coverage: The Experience of Health Care Reform in the United States*, edited by Jessica Mulligan and Heide Castañeda, 102–25. New York: New York University Press.

Angrist, Misha. 2022. "A Different Kind of 'Hangry.'" *Public Health Watch*, June 16, 2022. https://publichealthwatch.org.

Aouache, Rajaa, Louise Biquard, Daniel Vaiman, and Francisco Miralles. 2018. "Oxidative Stress in Preeclampsia and Placental Diseases." *International Journal of Molecular Sciences* 19 (5): 1496.

Artiga, Samantha, and Maria Diaz. 2019. *Health Coverage and Care of Undocumented Immigrants*. Kaiser Family Foundation, July 15, 2019. www.kff.org.

Assistant Secretary for Planning and Evaluation (ASPE). 2022. *Impact of the COVID-19 Pandemic on the Hospital and Outpatient Clinician Workforce: Challenges and Policy Responses*. US Department of Health and Human Services (Washington, DC). https://aspe.hhs.gov.

Aufdenblatten, Myriam, Marc Baumann, Luigi Raio, Bernhard Dick, Brigitte Frey, Henning Schneider, Daniel Surbek, Berthold Hocher, and Markus Mohaupt. 2009. "Prematurity is Related to High Placental Cortisol in Preeclampsia." *Pediatric Research* 65 (2): 198–202.

Baker, Mary, Yvonne Butler-Tobah, Abimbola Famuyide, and Regan Theiler. 2021. "Medicaid Cost and Reimbursement for Low-Risk Prenatal Care in the United States." *Journal of Midwifery and Women's Health* 66 (5): 589–96.

Balderrama, Francisco, and Raymond Rodríguez. 2006. *Decade of Betrayal: Mexican Repatriation in the 1930s*. Albuquerque: University of New Mexico Press.

Barofsky, Jeremy, Ariadna Vargas, Dinardo Rodriguez, and Anthony Barrows. 2020. "Spreading Fear: The Announcement of the Public Charge Rule Reduced Enrollment in Child Safety-Net Programs." *Health Affairs* 39 (10): 1752–61.

Barrios, Roberto. 2016. "Resilience: A Commentary from the Vantage Point of Anthropology." *Annals of Anthropological Practice* 40 (1): 28–38.

Bearblock, Elizabeth, Catherine Aiken, and Graham Burton. 2021. "Air Pollution and Pre-eclampsia: Associations and Potential Mechanisms." *Placenta* 104:188–94.

Beauvais, Sally, and Mitchell Ferman. 2021. "Texas' Unemployment System is Confusing and Frustrating. Here's How to Navigate It." *Texas Tribune*, June 30, 2021. https://www.texastribune.org.

Bhattacharya, Oashe, Bodrun Naher Siddiquea, Aishwarya Shetty, Afsana Afroz, and Baki Billah. 2022. "COVID-19 Vaccine Hesitancy among Pregnant Women: A Systematic Review and Meta-analysis." *BMJ Open* 12 (8): e061477.

Bibbins-Domingo, Kirsten, David Grossman, Susan Curry, Michael Barry, Karina Davidson, Chyke Doubeni, John Epling, Alex Kemper, Alex Krist, and Ann Kurth. 2017. "Screening for Preeclampsia: US Preventive Services Task Force Recommendation Statement." *Journal of the American Medical Association* 317 (16): 1661–7.

Bigelow, Catherine, Guilherme Pereira, Amber Warmsley, Jennifer Cohen, Chloe Getrajdman, Erin Moshier, Julia Paris, Angela Bianco, Stephanie Factor, and Joanne

Stone. 2014. "Risk Factors for New-Onset Late Postpartum Preeclampsia in Women without a History of Preeclampsia." *American Journal of Obstetrics and Gynecology* 210 (4): 338e1–338e8.

Bingham, Debra, Nan Strauss, and Francine Coeytaux. 2011. "Maternal Mortality in the United States: A Human Rights Failure." *Contraception* 83 (3): 189–93.

Boehm, Deborah. 2005. "The Safety Net of the Safety Net: How Federally Qualified Health Centers 'Subsidize' Medicaid Managed Care." *Medical Anthropology Quarterly* 19 (1): 47–63.

———. 2012. *Intimate Migrations: Gender, Family, and Illegality among Transnational Mexicans*. New York: New York University Press.

Bohn, Sarah, and Julien Lafortune. 2022. "Starting the Year with Less (Real) Money." *Public Policy Institute of California* (blog). www.ppic.org.

Bonaparte, Alicia. 2015. "Regulating Childbirth: Physicians and Granny Midwives in South Carolina." In *Birthing Justice: Black Women, Pregnancy, and Childbirth*, edited by Alicia Bonaparte and Julia Chinyere Oparah, 24–33. New York: Routledge.

Bourgois, Philippe. 1988. "Conjugated Oppression: Class and Ethnicity among Guaymi and Kuna Banana Workers." *American Ethnologist* 15 (2): 328–48.

Boylan, Peter, Peter O'Donovan, and Owen Owens. 1985. "Fetal Breathing Movements and the Diagnosis of Labor: A Prospective Analysis of 100 Cases." *Obstetrics and Gynecology* 66 (4): 517–20.

Brender, Jean, Lucina Suarez, Katherine Hendricks, Rich Ann Baetz, and Russell Larsen. 2002. "Parental Occupation and Neural Tube Defect-affected Pregnancies among Mexican Americans." *Journal of Occupational and Environmental Medicine* 44 (7): 650–6.

Bridges, Khiara. 2011. *Reproducing Race: An Ethnography of Pregnancy as a Site of Racialization*. Berkeley: University of California Press.

Brotherton, Sean, and Vinh-Kim Nguyen. 2013. "Revisiting Local Biology in the Era of Global Health." *Medical Anthropology* 32 (4): 287–90.

Buettgens, Matthew, Linda Blumberg, and Clare Pan. 2018. *The Uninsured in Texas: Statewide and Local Area Views*. Urban Institute, December 12, 2018. www.urban.org.

Callaghan, Timothy, David Washburn, Katharine Nimmons, Delia Duchicela, Anoop Gurram, and James Burdine. 2019. "Immigrant Health Access in Texas: Policy, Rhetoric, and Fear in the Trump Era." *BMC Health Services Research* 19 (1): 1–8.

Calvo Aguilar, Omar, Marta Torres Falcón, and Rosario Valdez Santiago. 2020. "Obstetric Violence Criminalised in Mexico: A Comparative Analysis of Hospital Complaints Filed with the Medical Arbitration Commission." *BMJ Sexual and Reproductive Health* 46 (1): 38–45.

Campbell, Howard. 2010. *Drug War Zone: Frontline Dispatches from the Streets of El Paso and Juárez*. Austin: University of Texas Press.

Campbell, Jana, and Ulrike Ehlert. 2012. "Acute Psychosocial Stress: Does the Emotional Stress Response Correspond with Physiological Responses?" *Psychoneuroendocrinology* 37 (8): 1111–34.

Carr, Eve Ariel. 2003. "Missionaries and Motherhood: Sixty-Six Years of Public Health Work in South El Paso." PhD, Department of History, Arizona State University.
Cartwright, Elizabeth. 2011. "Immigrant Dreams: Legal Pathologies and Structural Vulnerabilities Along the Immigration Continuum." *Medical Anthropology* 30 (5): 475–95.
Castañeda, Heide. 2018. "Stratification by Immigration Status: Contradictory Exclusion and Inclusion after Health Care Reform." In *Unequal Coverage: The Experience of Health Care Reform in the United States*, edited by Jessica Mulligan and Heide Castañeda, 35–58. New York: New York University Press.
———. 2019. *Borders of Belonging: Struggle and Solidarity in Mixed-Status Immigrant Families*. Redwood City, CA: Stanford University Press.
Castro, Arachu. 2019. "Witnessing Obstetric Violence during Fieldwork: Notes from Latin America." *Health and Human Rights* 21 (1): 103–11.
Castro, Arachu, and Virginia Savage. 2019. "Obstetric Violence as Reproductive Governance in the Dominican Republic." *Medical Anthropology* 38 (2): 123–36.
Castro, Roberto, and Joaquina Erviti. 2014. "25 Años de Investigación Sobre Violencia Obstétrica en México." *Revista Conamed* 19 (1): 37–42.
Cañas, Jesus, Pia Orrenius, and Juliette Coia. 2022. "Federal Aid Helps Border Keep Pace with Texas Economy during Pandemic Turmoil." Federal Reserve Bank of Dallas, March 1, 2022. www.dallasfed.org.
Center on Budget and Policy Priorities. 2023. "Chart Book: Tracking the Recovery from the Pandemic Recession." Last updated December 14, 2023. www.cbpp.org.
Centers for Disease Control and Prevention (CDC). 2023. "Percentage of Mothers with Gestational Diabetes by Maternal Age." *Morbidity and Mortality Weekly Report* 72 (16).
Cerdeña, Jessica. 2023. *Pressing Onward: The Imperative Resilience of Latina Migrant Mothers*. Berkeley: University of California Press.
Cerón-Becerra, Miguel. 2022. "Mistreatment of Pregnant Women in US Immigration Detention." *Blog of the American Philosophical Association* (blog), March 7, 2022. blog.apaonline.org.
Cerón-Mireles, Prudencia. 2006. "Detection and Risk Factors for Preeclampsia." PhD, Epidemiological Science, University of Michigan.
Chadwick, Rachelle, and Jabulile Mary-Jane Jace Mavuso. 2021. "On Reproductive Violence: Framing Notes." *Agenda* 35 (3): 1–11.
Chatterjee, Paula, Mingyu Qi, and Rachel Werner. 2021. "Association of Medicaid Expansion with Quality in Safety-Net Hospitals." *JAMA Internal Medicine* 181 (5): 590–7.
Chavez, Leo. 2008. *The Latino Threat: Constructing Immigrants, Citizens, and the Nation*. Redwood City, CA: Stanford University Press.
———. 2017. *Anchor Babies and the Challenge of Birthright Citizenship*. Redwood City, CA: Stanford University Press.
Chen, Jarvis, and Nancy Krieger. 2021. "Revealing the Unequal Burden of COVID-19 by Income, Race/Ethnicity, and Household Crowding: US County versus Zip Code Analyses." *Journal of Public Health Management and Practice* 27 (1): S43–56.

Chicoine, Luke. 2016. "Homicides in Mexico and the Expiration of the US Federal Assault Weapons Ban: A Difference-in-Discontinuities Approach." *Journal of Economic Geography* 17 (4): 825–56.

Cleek, Hailey. 2019. "Borders Across Bodies: Assessing the Balance of Expanding CHIP Coverage at the Expense of Advancing Fetal Personhood." *Berkeley Journal of Gender, Law, and Justice* 34:1–28.

Cloud, David, Cyrus Ahalt, Dallas Augustine, David Sears, and Brie Williams. 2020. "Medical Isolation and Solitary Confinement: Balancing Health and Humanity in US Jails and Prisons during COVID-19." *Journal of General Internal Medicine* 35 (9): 2738–42.

Conner, Phillip. 2021. *Immigration Reform Can Keep Millions of Mixed-Status Families Together*. FWD.us, September 9, 2021. www.fwd.us.

Cooper Owens, Deirdre. 2017. *Medical Bondage: Race, Gender, and the Origins of American Gynecology*. Athens: University of Georgia Press.

Coronado-Arroyo, Julia Cristina, Marcio José Concepción-Zavaleta, Francisca Elena Zavaleta-Gutiérrez, and Luis Alberto Concepción-Urteaga. 2021. "Is COVID-19 a Risk Factor for Severe Preeclampsia?: Hospital Experience in a Developing Country." *European Journal of Obstetrics, Gynecology, and Reproductive Biology* 256:502–3.

Crenshaw, Kimberlé. 1990. "Mapping the Margins: Intersectionality, Identity Politics, and Violence against Women of Color." *Stanford Law Review* 43:1241–300.

Csordas, Thomas. 1993. "Somatic Modes of Attention." *Cultural Anthropology* 8 (2): 135–56.

Daiber, Andreas, and Thomas Münzel. 2020. "Impact of Environmental Pollution and Stress on Redox Signaling and Oxidative Stress Pathways." *Redox Biology* 37:101621.

Dang, Bich Ngoc, Louise Van Dessel, June Hanke, and Margo Hilliard. 2011. "Birth Outcomes among Low-Income Women—Documented and Undocumented." *Permanente Journal* 15 (2): 39.

Das, Veena. 2004. "The Signature of the State: The Paradox of Illegibility." In *Anthropology and the Margins of the State*, edited by Veena Das and Deborah Poole, 225–52. Santa Fe, NM: School for Advanced Research Press.

Davies, Emma, Jacqueline Bell, and Sohinee Bhattacharya. 2016. "Preeclampsia and Preterm Delivery: A Population-Based Case-Control Study." *Hypertension in Pregnancy* 35 (4): 510–19.

Davis, Angela. 1983. *Women, Race, and Class*. New York: Knopf Doubleday.

Davis, Dána-Ain. 2019. *Reproductive Injustice: Racism, Pregnancy, and Premature Birth*. New York: New York University Press.

Davis-Floyd, Robbie. 1992. *Birth as an American Rite of Passage*. Berkeley: University of California Press.

Dawley, Katy. 2003. "Origins of Nurse-Midwifery in the United States and its Expansion in the 1940s." *Journal of Midwifery and Women's Health* 48 (2): 86–95.

De Anda, Victoria, and Carina Heckert. 2022. "Stratified Access to Care and Mental Health Implications for Pregnant and Postpartum Immigrants in the US-Mexico Border Region." In *Research Handbook on Society and Mental Health*, edited by Marta Elliott, 101–14. Cheltenham, UK: Edward Elgar.

De León, Jason. 2015. *Land of Open Graves: Living and Dying on the Migrant Trail*. Berkeley: University of California Press.

Declercq, Eugene, and Laurie Zephyrin. 2020. *Maternal Mortality in the United States: A Primer*. Commonwealth Fund, December 16, 2020. www.commonwealthfund.org.

Dehlendorf, Christine, Kira Levy, Rachel Ruskin, and Jody Steinauer. 2010. "Health Care Providers' Knowledge about Contraceptive Evidence: A Barrier to Quality Family Planning Care?" *Contraception* 81 (4): 292–8.

Dekker, Rebecca. 2019. *Evidence On: Induction for Gestational Diabetes*. Evidence Based Birth, last updated April 3, 2019. https://evidencebasedbirth.com.

Department of Homeland Security (DHS). 2023. *Fact Sheet: A Review by the Family Reunification Task Force on the Second Anniversary of Its Establishment*. DHS, February 2, 2023. www.dhs.gov.

Desjarlais, Robert, and Jason Throop. 2011. "Phenomenological Approaches in Anthropology." *Annual Review of Anthropology* 40:87–102.

Díaz-Barriga, Miguel, and Margaret Dorsey. 2020. *Fencing in Democracy: Border Walls, Necrocitizenship, and the Security State*. Durham, NC: Duke University Press.

Diaz-Tello, Farah. 2016. "Invisible Wounds: Obstetric Violence in the United States." *Reproductive Health Matters* 24 (47): 56–64.

Dickerson, Caitlin, and Michael Shear. 2020. "Before COVID-19, Trump Aide Sought to Use Disease to Close Borders." *New York Times*, May 3, 2020. www.nytimes.com.

Dixon, Lydia. 2015. "Obstetrics in a Time of Violence: Mexican Midwives Critique Routine Hospital Practices." *Medical Anthropology Quarterly* 29 (4): 437–54.

Dolin, Cara, Charlene Compher, Jinhee Oh, and Celeste Durnwald. 2021. "Pregnant and Hungry: Addressing Food Insecurity in Pregnant Women during the COVID-19 Pandemic in the United States." *American Journal of Obstetrics and Gynecology* 3 (4): 100378.

Donovan, Megan. 2018. "Self-Managed Medication Abortion: Expanding the Available Options for US Abortion Care." *Guttmacher Policy Review* 21: 41–47.

Downey, Greg. 2014. "'Habitus in Extremis': From Embodied Culture to Bio-cultural Development." *Body and Society* 20 (2): 113–7.

Dreby, Joanna. 2015. "US Immigration Policy and Family Separation: The Consequences for Children's Well-Being." *Social Science and Medicine* 132:245–51.

Dunkel Schetter, Christine, and Laura Glynn. 2011. "Stress in Pregnancy: Empirical Evidence and Theoretical Frameworks to Guide Interdisciplinary Research." In *The Handbook of Stress Science*, edited by Richard Contrada and Andrew Baum, 320–43. New York: Springer.

Dursun, Bahadir. 2019. "The Intergenerational Effects of Mass Shootings." *Social Science Research Network*. https://dx.doi.org/10.2139/ssrn.3474544.

Eichner, Maxine. 2022. "COVID-19 and the Perils of Free-Market Parenting: Why It Is Past Time for the United States to Install Government Supports for Families." *Fordham Law Review* 90 (6): 2509–28.

El Paso Health. 2022. *CHIP Perinatal Member Handbook*. elpasohealth.com.

El Paso Strong. 2020. "COVID-19 Reports." elpasostrong.com.

El Pasoans Fighting Hunger. 2023. "About Us." elpasoansfightinghunger.org.

Ellwood, Marilyn Rymer, and Genevieve Kenney. 1995. "Medicaid and Pregnant Women: Who is Being Enrolled and When." *Health Care Financing Review* 17 (2): 7–28.

Eskild, Anne, and Lars Vatten. 2009. "Abnormal Bleeding Associated with Preeclampsia: A Population Study of 315,085 Pregnancies." *Acta Obstetricia et Gynecologica Scandinavica* 88 (2): 154–8.

Fabi, Rachel. 2019. "Why Physicians Should Advocate for Undocumented Immigrants' Unimpeded Access to Prenatal Care." *AMA Journal of Ethics* 21 (1): 93–99.

Farfán-Santos, Elizabeth. 2019. "Undocumented Motherhood: Gender, Maternal Identity, and the Politics of Health Care." *Medical Anthropology* 38 (6): 523–36.

Farmer, Paul. 2003. *Pathologies of Power: Health, Human Rights, and the New War on the Poor*. Berkeley: University of California Press.

Fasanya, Henrietta, Chu Hsiao, Kendra Armstrong-Sylvester, and Stacy Beal. 2021. "A Critical Review on the Use of Race in Understanding Racial Disparities in Preeclampsia." *Journal of Applied Laboratory Medicine* 6 (1): 247–56.

Finkler, Kaja. 1994. *Women in Pain: Gender and Morbidity in Mexico*. Philadelphia: University of Pennsylvania Press.

Fisher-Hoch, Susan, Anne Rentfro, Gaines Wilson, Jennifer Salinas, Belinda Reininger, Blanca Restrepo, Joseph McCormick, et al. 2010. "Socioeconomic Status and Prevalence of Obesity and Diabetes in a Mexican American Community, Cameron County, Texas, 2004–2007." *Preventing Chronic Disease* 7 (3): A53.

Fleuriet, Jill, and Thankam Sunil. 2015. "Reproductive Habitus, Psychosocial Health, and Birth Weight Variation in Mexican Immigrant and Mexican American Women in South Texas." *Social Science and Medicine* 138:102–9.

———. 2017. "Stress, Pregnancy, and Motherhood: Implications for Birth Weights in the Borderlands of Texas." *Medical Anthropology Quarterly* 31 (1): 60–77.

Frederick, Angela. 2017. "Risky Mothers and the Normalcy Project: Women with Disabilities Negotiate Scientific Motherhood." *Gender and Society* 31 (1): 74–95.

Fuentes, César, and Sergio Peña. 2010. "Globalization, Transborder Networks, and US-Mexico Border Cities." In *Cities and Citizenship at the US-Mexico Border: The Paso del Norte Metropolitan Region*, edited by Kathleen Staudt, César Fuentes, and Julia Monárrez Fragoso, 1–19. New York: Palgrave Macmillan.

Fujita, Shigeru. 2022. "Labor Market Recovery during the COVID-19 Pandemic." *Economic Insights* 7 (2): 2–10.

Gálvez, Alyshia. 2011. *Patient Citizens, Immigrant Mothers: Mexican Women, Public Prenatal Care, and the Birth Weight Paradox*. New Brunswick, NJ: Rutgers University Press.

———. 2019. "Transnational Mother Blame: Protecting and Caring in a Globalized Context." *Medical Anthropology* 38 (7): 574–87.

Gereffi, Gary. 2018. "Mexico's 'Old' and 'New' Maquiladora Industries: Contrasting Approaches to North American Integration." In *Neoliberalism Revisited: Economic*

Restructuring and Mexico's Political Future, edited by Gerardo Otero, 85–105. New York: Routledge.
Geronimus, Arline. 1992. "The Weathering Hypothesis and the Health of African-American Women and Infants: Evidence and Speculations." *Ethnicity and Disease* 2 (3): 207–21.
Ghulmiyyah, Labib, and Baha Sibai. 2012. "Maternal Mortality from Preeclampsia/Eclampsia." *Seminars in Perinatology* 36 (1): 56–59.
Golash-Boza, Tanya, and Pierrette Hondagneu-Sotelo. 2013. "Latino Immigrant Men and the Deportation Crisis: A Gendered Racial Removal Program." *Latino Studies* 11 (3): 271–92.
Gómez Cervantes, Andrea, and Cecilia Menjívar. 2020. "Legal Violence, Health, and Access to Care: Latina Immigrants in Rural and Urban Kansas." *Journal of Health and Social Behavior* 61 (3): 307–23.
Gong, Jian, David Savitz, Cheryl Stein, and Stephanie Engel. 2012. "Maternal Ethnicity and Pre-eclampsia in New York City, 1995–2003." *Paediatric and Perinatal Epidemiology* 26 (1): 45–52.
Goodwin, Michele. 2020. *Policing the Womb: Invisible Women and the Criminalization of Motherhood*. Cambridge, UK: Cambridge University Press.
Goyal, Manu, Pratibha Singh, Kuldeep Singh, Shashank Shekhar, Neha Agrawal, and Sanjeev Misra. 2021. "The Effect of the COVID-19 Pandemic on Maternal Health Due to Delay in Seeking Health Care: Experience from a Tertiary Center." *International Journal of Gynecology and Obstetrics* 152 (2): 231–5.
Gravlee, Clarence. 2009. "How Race Becomes Biology: Embodiment of Social Inequality." *American Journal of Physical Anthropology* 139 (1): 47–57.
Grineski, Sara, and Patricia Juárez-Carrillo. 2012. "Environmental Injustice in the US-Mexico Border Region." In *Social Justice in the US-Mexico Border Region*, edited by Mark Lusk, Kathleen Staudt, and Eva Moya, 179–98. New York: Springer.
Gruber, Kenneth, Susan Cupito, and Christina Dobson. 2013. "Impact of Doulas on Healthy Birth Outcomes." *Journal of Perinatal Education* 22 (1): 49–58.
Grünebaum, Amos, Laurence McCullough, Risa Klein, and Frank Chervenak. 2020. "US Midwife-Attended Hospital Births are Increasing while Physician-Attended Hospital Births are Decreasing: 2003–2018." *American Journal of Obstetrics and Gynecology* 223 (3): 460–1.
Guarnaccia, Peter. 1993. "*Ataques de Nervios* in Puerto Rico: Culture-Bound Syndrome or Popular Illness?" *Medical Anthropology* 15 (2): 157–70.
Guarnaccia, Peter, and Pablo Farias. 1988. "The Social Meanings of *Nervios*: A Case Study of a Central American Woman." *Social Science and Medicine* 26 (12): 1223–31.
Gutierrez, Carmen, and Nathan Dollar. 2023. "Birth and Prenatal Care Outcomes of Latina Mothers in the Trump Era: Analysis by Nativity and Country/Region of Origin." *PLoS One* 18 (3): e0281803.
Gutiérrez, Elena. 2008. *Fertile Matters: The Politics of Mexican-Origin Women's Reproduction*. Austin: University of Texas Press.

Gutiérrez, Elena, and Liza Fuentes. 2009. "Population Control by Sterilization: The Cases of Puerto Rican and Mexican-Origin Women in the United States." *Latino(a) Research Review* 7 (3): 85–100.

Hampton, Elaine, and Cynthia Ontiveros. 2019. *Copper Stain: ASARCO's Legacy in El Paso.* Norman, OK: University of Oklahoma Press.

Haque, Omar Sultan, and Adam Waytz. 2012. "Dehumanization in Medicine: Causes, Solutions, and Functions." *Perspectives on Psychological Science* 7 (2): 176–86.

Hatzenbuehler, Mark, Seth Prins, Morgan Flake, Morgan Philbin, Somjen Frazer, Daniel Hagen, and Jennifer Hirsch. 2017. "Immigration Policies and Mental Health Morbidity among Latinos: A State-Level Analysis." *Social Science and Medicine* 174:169–78.

Hauspurg, Alisse, and Arun Jeyabalan. 2022. "Postpartum Preeclampsia or Eclampsia: Defining its Place and Management among the Hypertensive Disorders of Pregnancy." *American Journal of Obstetrics and Gynecology* 226 (2): S1211–21.

Have My Baby in Miami. 2021. "International Maternity Service of Miami." havemybabyinmiami.com.

Health Resources and Services Administration (HRSA). 2023. "MUA Find: Medically Underserved Area and Medically Underserved Population Designations." US Department of Health and Human Services. data.hrsa.gov.

Heckert, Carina. 2016. "When Care is a 'Systematic Route of Torture': Conceptualizing the Violence of Medical Negligence in Resource-Poor Settings." *Culture, Medicine, and Psychiatry* 40 (4): 687–706.

———. 2020. "The Bureaucratic Violence of the Health Care System for Pregnant Immigrants on the United States-Mexico Border." *Human Organization* 79 (1): 33–42.

Heckert, Carina, and Andrea Daniella Mata. Under review. "Stratified Access and Experiences of Maternal Health Care in the US-Mexico Border Region."

Hernandez, Emily, and Kalley Huang. 2022. "Families are Desperate for Child Care, but Providers Face a 'Roller Coaster' Trying to Survive." *Texas Tribune*, March 15, 2022. www.texastribune.org.

Hernández, Leandra, and Sarah De Los Santos Upton. 2019. "Critical Health Communication Methods at the US-Mexico Border: Violence against Migrant Women and the Role of Health Activism." *Frontiers in Communication* 4:34.

Heyman, Josiah. 2023. "The US-Mexico Border as a Model for Social-cultural Theory: A Brief Discussion." *City and Society* 35 (1): 8–13.

Heyman, Josiah, and Jeremy Slack. 2023. "The Causes behind the Ciudad Juárez Migrant Detention Center Fire." *North American Congress on Latin America Report*, April 20, 2023. https://nacla.org.

Hinton, Alexander. 1999. "Introduction." In *Biocultural Approaches to the Emotions*, edited by Alexander Hinton, 1–37. Cambridge, UK: Cambridge University Press.

Ho, Jui, John Lewis, Peter O'Loughlin, Christopher Bagley, Roberto Romero, Gus Dekker, and David Torpy. 2007. "Reduced Maternal Corticosteroid-binding Globulin and Cortisol Levels in Pre-eclampsia and Gamete Recipient Pregnancies." *Clinical Endocrinology* 66 (6): 869–77.

Holpuch, Amanda. 2020. "The 'Shecession': Why Economic Crisis is Affecting Women More than Men." *Guardian*, August 4, 2020. www.theguardian.com.

Horton, Sarah. 2016. *They Leave Their Kidneys in the Fields: Illness, Injury, and Illegality among US Farmworkers*. Berkeley: University of California Press.

———. 2022. "Praying for More Time: Mexican Immigrants' Pandemic Eldercare Dilemmas." *Medical Anthropology Quarterly* 36 (4): 497–514.

Horton, Sarah, and Judith Barker. 2016. "Embodied Inequalities: An Interdisciplinary Conversation on Oral Health Disparities." In *Understanding Health Inequalities and Justice: New Conversations across the Disciplines*, edited by Mara Buchbinder, Michele Rivkin-Fish, and Rebecca Walker, 137–59. Chapel Hill: University of North Carolina Press.

Horton, Sarah, Whitney Duncan, and Kristin Yarris. 2018. "Immigrant Communities and the Public Charge Rule." *Anthropology News* 59 (5).

Hummer, Robert, Daniel Powers, Starling Pullum, Ginger Gossman, and Parker Frisbie. 2007. "Paradox Found (Again): Infant Mortality among the Mexican-Origin Population in the United States." *Demography* 44 (3): 441–57.

Jayasuriya, Nimesh, Alice Hughes, Ulla Sovio, Emma Cook, Stephen Charnock-Jones, and Gordon Smith. 2019. "A Lower Maternal Cortisol-to-Cortisone Ratio Precedes Clinical Diagnosis of Preterm and Term Preeclampsia by Many Weeks." *Journal of Clinical Endocrinology and Metabolism* 104 (6): 2355–66.

Johnson, Jasmin, and Judette Louis. 2022. "Does Race or Ethnicity Play a Role in the Origin, Pathophysiology, and Outcomes of Preeclampsia?: An Expert Review of the Literature." *American Journal of Obstetrics and Gynecology* 226 (2): S876–85.

Kaiser Family Foundation (KFF). 2023. "State-Funded Health Coverage for Immigrants as of July 2023." KFF, July 26, 2023. www.kff.org.

Kladzyk, Rene. 2020. "El Paso Job Losses Disproportionately Impact Women, Young People." *El Paso Matters*, May 21, 2020. https://elpasomatters.org.

Kladzyk, Rene, Phil Galewitz, and Elizabeth Lucas. 2021. "Why COVID-19 Killed Texas Border Residents in Shocking Numbers." *El Paso Matters*, June 22, 2021. https://elpasomatters.org.

Kleinman, Arthur, and Peter Benson. 2006. "Anthropology in the Clinic: The Problem of Cultural Competency and How to Fix It." *PLoS Medicine* 3 (10): e294.

Kleinman, Arthur, Leon Eisenberg, and Byron Good. 1978. "Culture, Illness, and Care: Clinical Lessons from Anthropologic and Cross-Cultural Research." *Annals of Internal Medicine* 88 (2): 251–8.

Kornfeind, Katelin, and Heather Sipsma. 2018. "Exploring the Link between Maternity Leave and Postpartum Depression." *Women's Health Issues* 28 (4): 321–6.

Koumouitzes-Douvia, Jodi, and Catherine Carr. 2006. "Women's Perceptions of their Doula Support." *Journal of Perinatal Education* 15 (4): 34.

Krieger, Nancy. 2016. "Living and Dying at the Crossroads: Racism, Embodiment, and Why Theory Is Essential for a Public Health of Consequence." *American Journal of Public Health* 106 (5): 832–3.

Krieger, Nancy, and George Davey Smith. 2004. "Bodies Count and Body Counts: Social Epidemiology and Embodying Inequality." *Epidemiologic Reviews* 26 (1): 92–103.

Krieger, Nancy, Mary Huynh, Wenhui Li, Pamela Waterman, and Gretchen Van Wye. 2018. "Severe Sociopolitical Stressors and Preterm Births in New York City: 1 September 2015 to 31 August 2017." *Journal of Epidemiology and Community Health* 72 (12): 1147–52.

Kuzawa, Christopher, and Elizabeth Sweet. 2009. "Epigenetics and the Embodiment of Race: Developmental Origins of US Racial Disparities in Cardiovascular Health." *American Journal of Human Biology* 21 (1): 2–15.

Laster Pirtle, Whitney, and Tashelle Wright. 2021. "Structural Gendered Racism Revealed in Pandemic Times: Intersectional Approaches to Understanding Race and Gender Health Inequities in COVID-19." *Gender and Society* 35 (2): 168–79.

Laverty, Ciara, and Dieneke de Vos. 2021. "Reproductive Violence as a Category of Analysis: Disentangling the Relationship between 'the Sexual' and 'the Reproductive' in Transitional Justice." *International Journal of Transitional Justice* 15 (3): 616–35.

Lazarus, Richard. 1999. "Evolution of a Model of Stress, Coping, and Discrete Emotions." In *Handbook of Stress, Coping and Health, Implications for Nursing Research, Theory, and Practice*, edited by Virginia Hill Rice, 199–225. Thousand Oaks, CA: Sage.

Lee, Seung Mi, Roberto Romero, You Jeong Lee, In Sook Park, Chan-Wook Park, and Bo Hyun Yoon. 2012. "Systemic Inflammatory Stimulation by Microparticles Derived from Hypoxic Trophoblast as a Model for Inflammatory Response in Preeclampsia." *American Journal of Obstetrics and Gynecology* 207 (4): 337.e1–337.e8.

Lerner, Sharon. 2015. "The Real War on Families: Why the US Needs Paid Leave Now." *In These Times*, August 18, 2015. https://inthesetimes.com.

Li, Wen-Whai, Jeremy Sarnat, Amit Raysoni, Stefani Sarnat, Thomas Stock, Fernando Holguin, Roby Greenwald, Hector Olvera, and Brent Johnson. 2011. *Characterization of Traffic Related Air Pollution in Elementary Schools and its Impact on Asthmatic Children in El Paso, Texas*. National Urban Air Toxin Research Center, Research Report (20).

Liese, Kylea, Robbie Davis-Floyd, Karie Stewart, and Melissa Cheyney. 2021. "Obstetric Iatrogenesis in the United States: The Spectrum of Unintentional Harm, Disrespect, Violence, and Abuse." *Anthropology and Medicine* 28 (2): 188–204.

Lira, Natalie, and Alexandra Minna Stern. 2014. "Mexican Americans and Eugenic Sterilization: Resisting Reproductive Injustice in California, 1920–1950." *Aztlán: A Journal of Chicano Studies* 39 (2): 9–34.

Lloyd, Cathy, Julie Smith, and Katie Weinger. 2005. "Stress and Diabetes: A Review of the Links." *Diabetes Spectrum* 18 (2): 121–27.

Lock, Margaret. 1993. "Cultivating the Body: Anthropology and Epistemologies of Bodily Practice and Knowledge." *Annual Review of Anthropology* 22 (1): 133–55.

———. 2017. "Recovering the Body." *Annual Review of Anthropology* 46:1–14.

López, Iris. 2008. *Matters of Choice: Puerto Rican Women's Struggle for Reproductive Freedom.* New Brunswick, NJ: Rutgers University Press.
Lopez, William. 2019. *Separated: Family and Community in the Aftermath of an Immigration Raid.* Baltimore, MD: Johns Hopkins University Press.
Lopez, William, Daniel Kruger, Jorge Delva, Mikel Llanes, Charo Ledon, Adreanne Waller, Melanie Harner, Ramiro Martinez, Laura Sanders, Margaret Harner, and Barbara Israel. 2017. "Health Implications of an Immigration Raid: Findings from a Latino Community in the Midwestern United States." *Journal of Immigrant and Minority Health* 19 (3): 702–8.
Lucas, William, Heide Castañeda, and Milena Melo. 2023. "The Lingering Ache: Temporalities of Oral Health Suffering in United States-Mexico Border Communities." *Human Organization* 82 (2): 131–41.
MacDorman, Marian, Eugene Declercq, Howard Cabral, and Christine Morton. 2016. "Is the United States Maternal Mortality Rate Increasing? Disentangling Trends from Measurement Issues." *Obstetrics and Gynecology* 128 (3): 447–55.
MacDorman, Marian, Eugene Declercq, and Marie Thoma. 2018. "Trends in Texas Maternal Mortality by Maternal Age, Race/Ethnicity, and Cause of Death, 2006–2015." *Birth* 45 (2): 169–77.
MacDorman, Marian, and Gopal Singh. 1998. "Midwifery Care, Social and Medical Risk Factors, and Birth Outcomes in the USA." *Journal of Epidemiology and Community Health* 52 (5): 310–17.
MacDorman, Marian, Marie Thomas, Eugene Declcerq, and Elizabeth Howell. 2021. "Racial and Ethnic Disparities in Maternal Mortality in the United States Using Enhanced Vital Records, 2016–2017." *American Journal of Public Health* 111 (9): 1673–81.
Maldonado, Donna. 2022. "Family Disruptions and Maternal Health in COVID Times." MA thesis, Department of Sociology and Anthropology, University of Texas at El Paso.
Malmqvist, Ebba, Kristina Jakobsson, Håkan Tinnerberg, Anna Rignell-Hydbom, and Lars Rylander. 2013. "Gestational Diabetes and Preeclampsia in Association with Air Pollution at Levels below Current Air Quality Guidelines." *Environmental Health Perspectives* 121 (4): 488–93.
Marks, Kristin, Michael Whitaker, Nickolas Agathis, Onika Anglin, Jennifer Milucky, Kadam Patel, Huong Pham, Pam Daily Kirley, Breanna Kawasaki, and James Meek. 2022. "Hospitalization of Infants and Children Aged 0–4 Years with Laboratory-Confirmed COVID-19—COVID-NET, 14 States, March 2020–February 2022." *Morbidity and Mortality Weekly Report* 71 (11): 429–36.
Martínez, Rebecca. 2018. *Marked Women: The Cultural Politics of Cervical Cancer in Venezuela.* Redwood City, CA: Stanford University Press.
Martinez, Yoli, Christian McDonald, and Marina Starleaf Riker. 2020. "Database: C-Section and Episiotomy Rates in Texas Hospitals." *San Antonio Express-News*, December 3, 2020. www.expressnews.com.
Mathema, Silva. 2017. *State-by-State Estimates of the Family Members of Unauthorized Immigrants.* Center for American Progress, March 16, 2017. www.americanprogress.org.

Mattes, Dominik, and Claudia Lang. 2020. "Embodied Belonging: In/exclusion, Health Care, and Well-Being in a World in Motion." *Culture, Medicine, and Psychiatry* 45 (1): 2–21.

McCormack, Shannon Weeks. 2016. "Postpartum Taxation and the Squeezed Out Mom." *Georgetown Law Journal* 105: 1323–78.

McElwain, Colm, Eszter Tuboly, Fergus McCarthy, and Cathal McCarthy. 2020. "Mechanisms of Endothelial Dysfunction in Pre-eclampsia and Gestational Diabetes Mellitus: Windows into Future Cardiometabolic Health?" *Frontiers in Endocrinology* 11:1–19.

McKiernan-González, John. 2012. *Fevered Measures: Public Health and Race at the Texas-Mexico Border, 1848–1942*. Durham, NC: Duke University Press.

Meloni, Maurizio. 2015. "Epigenetics for the Social Sciences: Justice, Embodiment, and Inheritance in the Postgenomic Age." *New Genetics and Society* 34 (2): 125–51.

Mendoza, Manel, Itziar Garcia-Ruiz, Nerea Maiz, Carlota Rodo, Pablo Garcia-Manau, Berta Serrano, Rosa Maria Lopez-Martinez, Joan Balcells, Nuria Fernandez-Hidalgo, and Elena Carreras. 2020. "Pre-Eclampsia-Like Syndrome Induced by Severe COVID-19: A Prospective Observational Study." *BJOG: An International Journal of Obstetrics and Gynaecology* 127 (11): 1374–80.

Menjívar, Cecilia. 2006. "Liminal Legality: Salvadoran and Guatemalan Immigrants' Lives in the United States." *American Journal of Sociology* 11 (4): 999–1037.

Menjívar, Cecilia, and Leisy Abrego. 2012. "Legal Violence: Immigration Law and the Lives of Central American Immigrants." *American Journal of Sociology* 117 (5): 1380–421.

Messing, Ariella, Rachel Fabi, and Joanne Rosen. 2020. "Reproductive Injustice at the US Border." *American Journal of Public Health* 110 (3): 339–44.

Metzl, Jonathan, and Dorothy Roberts. 2014. "Structural Competency Meets Structural Racism: Race, Politics, and the Structure of Medical Knowledge." *AMA Journal of Ethics* 16 (9): 674–90.

Molina, Natalia. 2011. "Borders, Laborers, and Racialized Medicalization: Mexican Immigration and US Public Health Practices in the 20th Century." *American Journal of Public Health* 101 (6): 1024–31.

Moniz, Michelle, Kayte Spector-Bagdady, Michele Heisler, and Lisa Hope Harris. 2017. "Inpatient Postpartum Long-Acting Reversible Contraception: Care that Promotes Reproductive Justice." *Obstetrics and Gynecology* 130 (4): 783–7.

Montoya-Williams, Diana, Victoria Guazzelli Williamson, Michelle Cardel, Elena Fuentes-Afflick, Mildred Maldonado-Molina, and Lindsay Thompson. 2021. "The Hispanic/Latinx Perinatal Paradox in the United States: A Scoping Review and Recommendations to Guide Future Research." *Journal of Immigrant and Minority Health* 23 (5): 1078–91.

Morales, Maria Cristina. 2019. "The Manufacturing of the US-Mexico Border Crisis." In *The Oxford Handbook of Migration Crises*, edited by Cecilia Menjívar, Immanuel Ness and Marie Ruiz, 145–61. New York: Oxford University Press.

Morales, Maria Cristina, Pamela Prieto, and Cynthia Bejarano. 2014. "Transnational Entrepreneurs and Drug War Violence between Ciudad Juárez and El Paso." *Articulo: Journal of Urban Research* (10).

Moran-Thomas, Amy. 2019. *Traveling with Sugar: Chronicles of a Global Epidemic*. Berkeley: University of California Press.
Mullings, Leith, and Alaka Wali. 2001. *Stress and Resilience: The Social Context of Reproduction in Central Harlem*. New York: Kluwer Academic/Plenum Publishers.
Muñoz Martinez, Monica. 2018. *The Injustice Never Leaves You: Anti-Mexican Violence in Texas*. Cambridge, MA: Harvard University Press.
Murillo, Lina-Maria. 2016. "Birth Control on the Border: Race, Gender, Religion, and Class in the Making of the Birth Control Movement, El Paso, Texas, 1936–1973." PhD diss., Department of History, University of Texas at El Paso.
———. 2021. "Birth Control, Border Control: The Movement for Contraception in El Paso, Texas 1936–1940." *Pacific Historical Review* 90 (3): 314–44.
Nading, Alex. 2017. "Local Biologies, Leaky Things, and the Chemical Infrastructure of Global Health." *Medical Anthropology* 36 (2): 141–56.
Neal, Jeremy, Nicole Carlson, Julia Phillippi, Ellen Tilden, Denise Smith, Rachel Breman, Mary Dietrich, and Nancy Lowe. 2019. "Midwifery Presence in United States Medical Centers and Labor Care and Birth Outcomes among Low-Risk Nulliparous Women: A Consortium on Safe Labor Study." *Birth* 46 (3): 475–86.
Neel, Brian, and Robert Sargis. 2011. "The Paradox of Progress: Environmental Disruption of Metabolism and the Diabetes Epidemic." *Diabetes* 60 (7): 1838–48.
Nephew, Lauren. 2021. "Systemic Racism and Overcoming My COVID-19 Vaccine Hesitancy." *EClinicalMedicine* 32.
Ngai, Mae. 2006. "Birthright Citizenship and the Alien Citizen." *Fordham Law Review* 75: 2521–30.
Novak, Nicole, Arline Geronimus, and Aresha Martinez-Cardoso. 2017. "Change in Birth Outcomes among Infants Born to Latina Mothers after a Major Immigration Raid." *International Journal of Epidemiology* 46 (3): 839–49.
Núñez-Mchiri, Guillermina Gina, and Josiah Heyman. 2007. "Entrapment Processes and Immigrant Communities in a Time of Heightened Border Vigilance." *Human Organization* 66 (4): 354–65.
Núñez-Mchiri, Guillermina Gina, Diana Riviera, and Corina Marrufo. 2017. "Portraits of Food Insecurity in Colonias in the US-Mexico Border Region." In *The US-Mexico Transborder Region: Cultural Dynamics and Historical Interactions*, edited by Carlos Vélez-Ibáñez and Josiah Heyman, 342–69. Tucson: University of Arizona Press.
Oaks, Laury, and Barbara Herr Harthorn. 2003. "Health and the Social and Cultural Construction of Risk." In *Risk, Culture, and Health Inequality: Shifting Perceptions of Danger and Blame*, edited by Barbara Herr Harthorn and Laury Oaks, 3–12. Westport, CT: Praeger.
Organista, Kurt, Sonya Arreola, and Torsten Neilands. 2016. "*La Desesperación* in Latino Migrant Day Laborers and its Role in Alcohol and Substance-Related Sexual Risk." *Social Science and Medicine Population Health* 2:32–42.
Orraca, Pedro, David Rocha, and Eunice Vargas. 2017. "Cross-Border School Enrollment: Associated Factors in the US-Mexico Borderlands." *Social Science Journal* 54 (4): 389–402.

Ovalle, Michelle. 2020. "*¡Bienvenido! a El Segundo Barrio:* Inside a Border Town's Beloved Neighborhood." *Medium* (blog), December 13, 2020. https://medium.com.

Ovesen, Per Glud, Dorte Møller Jensen, Peter Damm, Steen Rasmussen, and Ulrik Schiøler Kesmodel. 2015. "Maternal and Neonatal Outcomes in Pregnancies Complicated by Gestational Diabetes: A Nation-wide Study." *Journal of Maternal-Fetal and Neonatal Medicine* 28 (14): 1720–24.

Papageorghiou, Aris, Philippe Deruelle, Robert Gunier, Stephen Rauch, Perla García-May, Mohak Mhatre, Mustapha Ado Usman, Sherief Abd-Elsalam, Saturday Etuk, and Lavone Simmons. 2021. "Preeclampsia and COVID-19: Results from the INTERCOVID Prospective Longitudinal Study." *American Journal of Obstetrics and Gynecology* 225 (3): 289.e1–289.e17.

Park, Lisa Sun-Hee. 2011. *Entitled to Nothing: The Struggle for Immigrant Health Care in the Age of Welfare Reform.* New York: New York University Press.

Parson, Nia, and Carina Heckert. 2014. "The Golden Cage: The Production of Insecurity at the Nexus of Intimate Partner Violence and Unauthorized Migration in the United States." *Human Organization* 73 (4): 305–14.

Patel, Divya, Salahuddin Meliha, Rose Gowen, Susan Fischer-Hoch, and Joseph McCormick. 2017. "Maternal Risk Factors in a Cohort Study of Mexican Americans Living Near the US-Mexico Border." *Obstetrics and Gynecology* 29 (5): S185–6.

Pathak, Arohi, Marc Jarsulic, and Osub Ahmed. 2022. *The National Baby Formula Shortage and the Inequitable US Food System.* Center for American Progress, June 17, 2022. www.americanprogress.org.

Pearson, Jennifer, Kale Siebert, Samantha Carlson, and Nathan Ratner. 2018. "Patient Perspectives on Loss of Local Obstetrical Services in Rural Northern Minnesota." *Birth* 45 (3): 286–94.

Pérez D'Gregorio, Rogelio. 2010. "Obstetric Violence: A New Legal Term Introduced in Venezuela." *Journal of Gynecology and Obstetrics* 111 (3): 201–2.

Philbin, Morgan, Morgan Flake, Mark Hatzenbuehler, and Jennifer Hirsch. 2017. "State-Level Immigration and Immigrant-Focused Policies as Drivers of Latino Health Disparities in the United States." *Social Science and Medicine* 199:29–38.

Piñeda, Richard. 2022. "Inconvenient Horror: Violence as Rhetoric and the El Paso Shooting." *Rhetoric and Public Affairs* 25 (3): 127–43.

Purkerson, Mabel, and Lilla Vekerdy. 1999. "A History of Eclampsia, Toxemia and the Kidney in Pregnancy." *American Journal of Nephrology* 19 (2): 313–9.

Pérez-Armendáriz, Clarisa. 2021. "Migrant Transnationalism in Violent Democracies." *Journal of Ethnic and Migration Studies* 47 (6): 1327–48.

Quesada, James. 2011. "'*No Soy Welferero*': Undocumented Latino Laborers in the Crosshairs of Legitimation Maneuvers." *Medical Anthropology* 30 (4): 386–408.

Quesada, James, Laurie Kain Hart, and Philippe Bourgois. 2011. "Structural Vulnerability and Health: Latino Migrant Laborers in the United States." *Medical Anthropology* 30 (4): 339–62.

Rad, Afagh Hassanzadeh, Gelayol Chatrnour, Samaneh Ghazanfar Tehran, and Amirhossein Fakhre Yaseri. 2022. "The Association between Preeclampsia and

COVID-19: A Narrative Review on Recent Findings." *Journal of Renal Injury Prevention* 11 (4): e32061.
Ramírez de Arellano, Annette, and Conrad Seipp. 2017. *Colonialism, Catholicism, and Contraception: A History of Birth Control in Puerto Rico*. Durham, NC: University of North Carolina Press.
Ranji, Usha, Brittni Frederiksen, Alina Salganicoff, and Michelle Long. 2021. *Women, Work, and Family During COVID-19: Findings from the KFF Women's Health Survey*. Kaiser Family Foundation, March 22, 2021. www.kff.org.
Redman, Christopher, and Ian Sargent. 2004. "Preeclampsia and the Systemic Inflammatory Response." *Seminars in Nephrology* 24 (6): 565–70.
Reed-Sandoval, Amy. 2022. "Border-Crossing for Abortion: A Feminist Challenge to Border Theory." *Journal of Social Philosophy* 53:296–316.
Rice, Kathleen. 2023. "Re-centering Relationships: Obstetric Violence, Health Care Rationalities, and Pandemic Childbirth in Canada." *Medical Anthropology Quarterly* 37 (1): 59–75.
Ríos, Viridiana. 2014. "Security Issues and Immigration Flows: Drug-Violence Refugees, the New Mexican Immigrants." *Latin American Research Review* 49 (3): 3.
Rivkin-Fish, Michele. 2013. "Conceptualizing Feminist Strategies for Russian Reproductive Politics: Abortion, Surrogate Motherhood, and Family Support after Socialism." *Signs* 38 (3): 569–93.
Roberts, Dorothy. 1997. *Killing the Black Body: Race, Reproduction, and the Meaning of Liberty*. New York: Vintage Books.
———. 2015. "Reproductive Justice, Not Just Rights." *Dissent* 62 (4): 79–82.
Roberts, James, and Mandy Bell. 2013. "If We Know So Much about Preeclampsia, Why Haven't We Cured the Disease?" *Journal of Reproductive Immunology* 99 (1–2): 1–9.
Roberts, James, Lisa Bodnar, Thelma Patrick, and Robert Powers. 2011. "The Role of Obesity in Preeclampsia." *Pregnancy Hypertension* 1 (1): 6–16.
Roberts, James, and Hilary Gammill. 2005. "Preeclampsia: Recent Insights." *Hypertension* 46 (6): 1243–9.
Robillard, Pierre-Yves, Gustaaf Dekker, Gérard Chaouat, Marco Scioscia, Silvia Iacobelli, and Thomas Hulsey. 2017. "Historical Evolution of Ideas on Eclampsia/Preeclampsia: A Proposed Optimistic View of Preeclampsia." *Journal of Reproductive Immunology* 123:72–77.
Robinson, Stephanie. 2017. "The Former Asarco Demolition Fallout: A Post Study on Lead Soil Concentrations and Environmental Agents of Redistribution in El Paso, TX." MS thesis, Department of Geology, University of Texas at El Paso.
Rodriguez, Maria, Jonas Swartz, Duncan Lawrence, and Aaron Caughey. 2020. "Extending Delivery Coverage to Include Prenatal Care for Low-Income, Immigrant Women is a Cost-Effective Strategy." *Women's Health Issues* 30 (4): 240–7.
Romo, David 2005. *Ringside Seat to a Revolution: An Underground Cultural History of El Paso and Juárez, 1893–1923*. El Paso, TX: Cinco Puntos Press.

Rooks, Judith. 1999. "The Midwifery Model of Care." *Journal of Nurse-Midwifery* 44 (4): 370–4.

Rosas, Gilberto. 2006. "The Managed Violences of the Borderlands: Treacherous Geographies, Policeability, and the Politics of Race." *Latino Studies* 4 (4): 401–18.

———. 2023. *Unsettling: The El Paso Massacre, Resurgent White Nationalism, and the US-Mexico Border*. Baltimore: Johns Hopkins University Press.

Rosen, Emma, Isabel Muñoz, Thomas McElrath, David Cantonwine, and Kelly Ferguson. 2018. "Environmental Contaminants and Preeclampsia: A Systematic Literature Review." *Journal of Toxicology and Environmental Health* 21 (5): 291–319.

Rosen, Jonathan, and Roberto Zepeda. 2016. *Organized Crime, Drug Trafficking, and Violence in Mexico: The Transition from Felipe Calderón to Enrique Peña Nieto*. Lanham, MD: Lexington Books.

Rosenthal, Lisa, and Marci Lobel. 2020. "Gendered Racism and the Sexual and Reproductive Health of Black and Latina Women." *Ethnicity and Health* 25 (3): 367–92.

Ross, Loretta. 2017. "Reproductive Justice as Intersectional Feminist Activism." *Souls* 19 (3): 286–314.

Russell, Evan, Gideo Koren, Michael Rieder, and Stan Van Uum. 2012. "Hair Cortisol as a Biological Marker of Chronic Stress: Current Status, Future Directions, and Unanswered Questions." *Psychoneuroendocrinology* 37 (5): 589–601.

Sabo, Samantha, Susan Shaw, Maia Ingram, Nicolette Teufel-Shone, Scott Carvajal, Jill Guernsey de Zapien, Cecilia Rosales, Flor Redondo, Gina Garcia, and Raquel Rubio-Goldsmith. 2014. "Everyday Violence, Structural Racism and Mistreatment at the US-Mexico Border." *Social Science and Medicine* 109:66–74.

Sadler, Michelle, Gonzalo Leiva, and Ibone Olza. 2020. "COVID-19 as a Risk Factor for Obstetric Violence." *Sexual and Reproductive Health Matters* 28 (1): 46–48.

Salcido, Olivia, and Madelaine Adelman. 2004. "'He Has Me Tied with the Blessed and Damned Papers': Undocumented Immigrant Battered Women in Phoenix, Arizona." *Human Organization* 63 (2): 162–72.

Saldaña-Tejeda, Abril. 2021. "'You Are Putting My Health at Risk': Genes, Diets and Bioethics under COVID-19 in Mexico." In *Viral Loads: Anthropologies of Urgency in the Time of COVID-19*, edited by Lenore Manderson, Nancy Burke, and Ayo Wahlberg, 260–80. London: University College London Press.

Samuels, Alex. 2020. "The Devastating Toll of COVID-19 on El Paso Illustrates the Pandemic's Stark Inequalities." *Texas Tribune*, November 21, 2020. www.texastribune.org.

Scragg, Anne Bacchini. 1981. "Problems in Professionalization of a Marginal Occupation: Midwifery in El Paso, Texas." MA thesis, Department of Sociology and Anthropology, University of Texas at El Paso.

Shah, Malika, and Ola Didrik Saugstad. 2021. "Newborns at Risk of Covid-19—Lessons from the Last Year." *Journal of Perinatal Medicine* 49 (6): 643–9.

Shashar, Sagi, Itai Kloog, Offer Erez, Alexandra Shtein, Maayan Yitshak-Sade, Batia Sarov, and Lena Novack. 2020. "Temperature and Preeclampsia: Epidemiological

Evidence that Perturbation in Maternal Heat Homeostasis affects Pregnancy Outcome." *PLoS One* 15 (5): e0232877.

Shen, Yun, Peng Wang, Leishen Wang, Shuang Zhang, Huikun Liu, Weiqin Li, Nan Li, Wei Li, Junhong Leng, and Jing Wang. 2018. "Gestational Diabetes with Diabetes and Prediabetes Risks: A Large Observational Study." *European Journal of Endocrinology* 179 (1): 51–58.

Sher, Lucien Derek, Hannah Geddie, Lukas Olivier, Megan Cairns, Nina Truter, Leandrie Beselaar, and Faadiel Essop. 2020. "Chronic Stress and Endothelial Dysfunction: Mechanisms, Experimental Challenges, and the Way Ahead." *American Journal of Physiology-Heart and Circulatory Physiology* 319 (2): H488–H506.

Sherman-Stokes, Sarah. 2021. "Public Health and the Power to Exclude: Immigrant Expulsions at the Border." *Georgetown Immigration Law Journal* 36:261–89.

Shih, Tiffany, Desi Peneva, Xiao Xu, Amelia Sutton, Elizabeth Triche, Richard Ehrenkranz, Michael Paidas, and Warren Stevens. 2016. "The Rising Burden of Preeclampsia in the United States Impacts both Maternal and Child Health." *American Journal of Perinatology* 33:329–38.

Shirk, David. 2010. "Drug Violence in Mexico: Data and Analysis from 2001–2009." *Trends in Organized Crime* 13 (2–3): 167–74.

Shojaei, Behnaz, Marzeyeh Loripoor, Mahmoud Sheikhfathollahi, and Fariba Aminzadeh. 2021. "The Effect of Walking during Late Pregnancy on the Outcomes of Labor and Delivery: A Randomized Clinical Trial." *Journal of Education and Health Promotion* 10 (277).

Siddaway, Andy, Peter Taylor, and Alex Wood. 2018. "Reconceptualizing Anxiety as a Continuum That Ranges from High Calmness to High Anxiety: The Joint Importance of Reducing Distress and Increasing Well-Being." *Journal of Personality and Social Psychology* 114 (2): e1–e11.

Sieff, Kevin. 2018. "U.S. Is Denying Passports to Americans along the Border, Throwing their Citizenship into Question." *Washington Post*, September 13, 2018. www.washingtonpost.com.

Sikkema, Marko, Pascale Robles de Medina, Roald Schaad, Edu Mulder, Hein Bruinse, Jan Buitelaar, Gerard Visser, and Arie Franx. 2001. "Salivary Cortisol Levels and Anxiety are Not Increased in Women Destined to Develop Preeclampsia." *Journal of Psychosomatic Research* 50 (1): 45–49.

Simpson, Kathleen Rice. 2022. "Trends in Labor Induction in the United States, 1989 to 2020." *MCN: The American Journal of Maternal/Child Nursing* 47 (4): 235.

Sinclair, Heather. 2016. "Birth City: Race and Violence in the History of Childbirth and Midwifery in the El Paso-Ciudad Juarez Borderlands, 1907–2013." PhD diss., Department of History, University of Texas at El Paso.

Singer, Merrill. 2009. *Introduction to Syndemics: A Critical and Systems Approach to Public and Community Health*. San Francisco, CA: Jossey-Bass.

Slack, Jeremy. 2019. *Deported to Death: How Drug Violence is Changing Migration on the US-Mexico Border*. Berkeley: University of California Press.

Smith-Oka, Vania. 2012. "Bodies of Risk: Constructing Motherhood in a Mexican Public Hospital." *Social Science and Medicine* 75 (12): 2275–82.

———. 2022. "Cutting Women: Unnecessary Cesareans as Iatrogenesis and Obstetric Violence." *Social Science and Medicine* 296:114734.

Solis, Isabela, and Carina Heckert. 2021. "Case Studies of Intimate Partner Violence, Immigration-Related Stress, and Legal Violence during Pregnancy in the US-Mexico Border Region." *Affilia* 36 (1): 27–42.

Soto, Gabriella, and Daniel Martínez. 2018. "The Geography of Migrant Death: Implications for Policy and Forensic Science." In *Sociopolitics of Migrant Death and Repatriation: Perspectives from Forensic Science*, edited by Alyson O'Daniel and Krista Latham, 67–82. New York: Springer.

Speer, Linda. 2019. "Misoprostol Alone is Associated with High Rate of Successful First-Trimester Abortion." *American Family Physician* 100 (2): 119.

Stephen, Lynn. 2007. *Transborder Lives: Indigenous Oaxacans in Mexico, California, and Oregon*. Durham, NC: Duke University Press.

Stockdale, Susan, Isabel Lagomasino, Juned Siddique, Thomas McGuire, and Jeanne Miranda. 2008. "Racial and Ethnic Disparities in Detection and Treatment of Depression and Anxiety among Psychiatric and Primary Health Care Visits, 1995–2005." *Medical Care* 46 (7): 668–77.

Strong, Adrienne. 2020. *Documenting Death: Maternal Mortality and the Ethics of Care in Tanzania*. Berkeley: University of California Press.

Suarez, Alicia. 2020. "Black Midwifery in the United States: Past, Present, and Future." *Sociology Compass* 14 (11): 1–12.

Suarez, Lucina, Marilyn Felkner, Jean Brender, Mark Canfield, Huiping Zhu, and Katherine Hendricks. 2012. "Neural Tube Defects on the Texas-Mexico Border: What We've Learned in the 20 Years since the Brownsville Cluster." *Clinical and Molecular Teratology* 94 (11): 882–92.

Tahir, Darius. 2019. "'Black Hole' of Medical Records Contributes to Death, Mistreatment at the Border." *Politico*, December 1, 2019. www.politico.com.

Takiuti, Nilton Hideto, Soubhi Kahhale, and Marcelo Zugaib. 2003. "Stress-Related Preeclampsia: An Evolutionary Maladaptation in Exaggerated Stress during Pregnancy?" *Medical Hypotheses* 60 (3): 328–31.

Talavera, Victor, Guillermina Gina Núñez-Mchiri, and Josiah Heyman. 2010. "Deportation in the US-Mexico Borderlands." In *The Deportation Regime: Sovereignty, Space, and the Freedom of Movement*, edited by Nicholas De Genova and Nathalie Peutz, 166–95. Durham, NC: Duke University Press.

Tapias, Maria. 2015. *Embodied Protests: Emotions and Women's Health in Bolivia*. Urbana: University of Illinois Press.

Texas Department of State Health Services (DSHS). 2018. *Maternal Mortality and Morbidity Task Force and Department of State Health Services Joint Biennial Report*. Texas Health and Human Services. www.hhs.texas.gov.

———. 2019. *External Quality Review of Texas Medicaid and CHIP Managed Care*. Texas Health and Human Services. www.hhs.texas.gov.

———. 2020. *External Quality Review of Texas Medicaid and CHIP Managed Care.* Texas Health and Human Services. www.hhs.texas.gov.

———. 2021. *External Quality Review of Texas Medicaid and CHIP Managed Care.* Texas Health and Human Services. www.hhs.texas.gov.

———. n.d. *Medicaid for the Elderly and People with Disabilities Handbook.* Texas Health and Human Services. www.hhs.texas.gov.

Texas Health and Human Services (HHS). 2022. *Texas Medicaid and CHIP Reference Guide.* Texas Health and Human Services Commission. www.hhs.texas.gov.

Texas Medical Association. 2016. "The Uninsured in Texas." Last updated November 13, 2019. www.texmed.org.

Torche, Florencia, and Catherine Sirois. 2019. "Restrictive Immigration Law and Birth Outcomes of Immigrant Women." *American Journal of Epidemiology* 188 (1): 24–33.

Uribarri, Laura Margarita. 2021. "Transboundary Air Quality Governance: A Case Study of the Paso Del Norte Air Basin 1940–2000." PhD diss., Department of History, University of Texas at El Paso.

US Census Bureau. 2021. "Quick Facts: El Paso County, Texas." www.census.gov.

US Department of State. 2022. *U.S. Relations with Mexico.* Bureau of Western Hemisphere Affairs, September 13, 2023. www.state.gov.

US Department of Transportation (DOT). 2017. "Border Crossing/Entry Data." Bureau of Transportation Statistics, last updated February 16, 2018. www.bts.gov.

Valdez, Natali, and Daisy Deomampo. 2019. "Centering Race and Racism in Reproduction." *Medical Anthropology* 38 (7): 551–9.

Van Esch, Joris, Antoinette Bolte, Frank Vandenbussche, Daniela Schippers, Carolina de Weerth, and Roseriet Beijers. 2020. "Differences in Hair Cortisol Concentrations and Reported Anxiety in Women with Preeclampsia versus Uncomplicated Pregnancies." *Pregnancy Hypertension* 21:200–2.

Vianna, Priscila, Moisés Bauer, Dinara Dornfeld, and José Artur Bogo Chies. 2011. "Distress Conditions during Pregnancy May Lead to Pre-Eclampsia by Increasing Cortisol Levels and Altering Lymphocyte Sensitivity to Glucocorticoids." *Medical Hypotheses* 77 (2): 188–91.

Vijayaraghavan, Maya, Guozhong He, Pamela Stoddard, and Dean Schillinger. 2010. "Blood Pressure Control, Hypertension, Awareness, and Treatment in Adults with Diabetes in the United States-Mexico Border Region." *Revista Panamericana de Salud Pública* 28 (3): 164–73.

Viladrich, Anahí. 2012. "Beyond Welfare Reform: Reframing Undocumented Immigrants' Entitlement to Health Care in the United States, a Critical Review." *Social Science and Medicine* 74 (6): 822–9.

Vogt, Wendy. 2017. "The Arterial Border: Negotiating Economies of Risk and Violence in Mexico's Security Regime." *International Journal of Migration and Border Studies* 3 (2–3): 192–207.

Von Dadelszen, Peter, and Laura Magee. 2014. "Pre-eclampsia: An Update." *Current Hypertension Reports* 16:1–14.

Vélez-Ibáñez, Carlos, and Josiah Heyman. 2017. *The US-Mexico Transborder Region: Cultural Dynamics and Historical Interactions.* Tucson: University of Arizona Press.

Vélez-Ibáñez, Carlos. 1980. "The Nonconsenting Sterilization of Mexican Women in Los Angeles: Issues of Psychocultural Rupture and Legal Redress in Paternalistic Behavioral Environments." In *Twice a Minority: Mexican American Women*, edited by Margarita Melville, 235–48. Maryland Heights, MO: Mosby Inc.

Wahlberg, Ayo, Nancy Burke, and Lenore Manderson. 2021. "Introduction: Stratified Livability and Pandemic Effects." In *Viral Loads: Anthropologies of Urgency in the Time of COVID-19*, edited by Lenore Manderson, Nancy Burke, and Ayo Wahlberg, 1–23. London: University College London Press.

Washington, Harriet. 2006. *Medical Apartheid: The Dark History of Medical Experimentation on Black Americans from Colonial Times to the Present.* New York: Doubleday Books.

Weech-Maldonado, Robert, Marc Elliott, Rohit Pradhan, Cameron Schiller, Janice Dreachslin, and Ron Hays. 2012. "Moving Towards Culturally Competent Health Systems: Organizational and Market Factors." *Social Science and Medicine* 75 (5): 815–22.

Willard, Keenan. 2020. "El Paso Moves to 10 Mobile Morgues for COVID-19 Deaths as Judge Wants to Extend Shutdown." *KFOX14*, November 9, 2020. https://kfoxtv.com.

Willen, Sarah. 2007. "Toward a Critical Phenomenology of 'Illegality': State Power, Criminalization, and Abjectivity among Undocumented Migrant Workers in Tel Aviv, Israel." *International Migration* 45 (3): 8–38.

———. 2012. "Migration, 'Illegality,' and Health: Mapping Embodied Vulnerability and Debating Health-Related Deservingness." *Social Science and Medicine* 74 (6): 805–11.

Williams, David, and Morgan Medlock. 2017. "Health Effects of Dramatic Societal Events—Ramifications of the Recent Presidential Election." *New England Journal of Medicine* 376 (23): 2295–9.

Williamson, Eliza. 2021. "The Iatrogenesis of Obstetric Racism in Brazil: Beyond the Body, Beyond the Clinic." *Anthropology and Medicine* 28 (2): 172–87.

Woolhandler, Steffie, David Himmelstein, Sameer Ahmed, Zinzi Bailey, Mary Bassett, Michael Bird, Jacob Bor, David Bor, Olveen Carrasquillo, and Merlin Chowkwanyun. 2021. "Public Policy and Health in the Trump Era." *Lancet* 397 (10275): 705–53.

Wosu, Adaeze, Unnur Valdimarsdóttir, Alexandra Shields, David Williams, and Michelle Williams. 2013. "Correlates of Cortisol in Human Hair: Implications for Epidemiologic Studies on Health Effects of Chronic Stress." *Annals of Epidemiology* 23 (12): 797–811.

Wright, Kathy, Jodi Ford, Joseph Perazzo, Lenette Jones, Sherrilynn Mahari, Brent Sullenbarger, and Mark Laudenslager. 2018. "Collecting Hair Samples for Hair Cortisol Analysis in African Americans." *Journal of Visualized Experiments* 136:e57288.

Wulsin, Lawson, Paul Horn, Jennifer Perry, Joseph Massaro, and Ralph D'Agostino. 2015. "Autonomic Imbalance as a Predictor of Metabolic Risks, Cardiovascular

Disease, Diabetes, and Mortality." *Journal of Clinical Endocrinology and Metabolism* 100 (6): 2443–8.

Yancey, Lynne, Elizabeth Withers, Katherine Bakes, and Jean Abbott. 2011. "Postpartum Preeclampsia: Emergency Department Presentation and Management." *Journal of Emergency Medicine* 40 (4): 380–4.

Yoder, Hannah, and Lynda Hardy. 2018. "Midwifery and Antenatal Care for Black Women: A Narrative Review." *SAGE Open* 8 (1).

Yu, Yunxian, Shanchun Zhang, Guoying Wang, Xiumei Hong, Eric Mallow, Sheila Walker, Colleen Pearson, Linda Heffner, Barry Zuckerman, and Xiaobin Wang. 2013. "The Combined Association of Psychosocial Stress and Chronic Hypertension with Preeclampsia." *American Journal of Obstetrics and Gynecology* 209 (5): 438.e1–438.e12.

Zanhour, Mona, and Dana McDaniel Sumpter. 2022. "The Entrenchment of the Ideal Worker Norm during the COVID-19 Pandemic: Evidence from Working Mothers in the United States." *Gender, Work, and Organization*, July 6, 2022.

Zavella, Patricia. 2020. *The Movement for Reproductive Justice: Empowering Women of Color through Social Activism*. New York: New York University Press.

Zhang, Shanchun, Zheyuan Ding, Hui Liu, Zexin Chen, Jinhua Wu, Youding Zhang, and Yunxian Yu. 2013. "Association between Mental Stress and Gestational Hypertension/Preeclampsia: A Meta-Analysis." *Obstetrical and Gynecological Survey* 68 (12): 825–34.

INDEX

Abbott, Greg, 25, 184, 213
abortion: decriminalization in Mexico, 62, 64; gestational limits, 63–64, 153; medicated, 63, 185; Texas abortion ban, 26, 63, 185; Texas Senate Bill 8 (SB-8), 63–64. *See also* Roe v. Wade
Abrego, Leisy, 29, 72
Adelaide, 56–58
Affordable Care Act (ACA), 7, 8, 187, 211n2
Aída, 82–83, 85, 87, 205
air pollution, 97–98, 108, 213n8
alien citizens, 12
Alma, 51, 172–74, 206, 214n11, 216n3
American Association of Obstetrics and Gynecology, 138
American College of Obstetrics and Gynecology, 91
American Medical Association, 10, 138
American Rescue Plan, 45, 103, 149, 215n1
American Smeltering and Refining Company (ASARCO), 97. *See also* environmental injustice
Anahí, 60, 70–72, 211n1
anchor baby, 12
Andaya, Elise, 8. *See also* temporary zone of inclusion
Anessa, 39–40, 42, 66, 76–77, 128–30, 146, 150–52, 159–60, 175, 207
Antebellum South, 138
anxiety: abuse, 84; COVID-19, 35, 121–26, 173, 206; *desesperación*, 3; economic, 6, 105, 169–70; immigration, 1, 4, 25, 28, 31, 32, 52, 74, 82, 87; mass shooting, 192, 207; medication, 104; preeclampsia's

link to, 99; pregnancy and birth, 83. *See also nervios*
asylum: international law, 13; seekers, 24, 181–184, 186, 190, 206, 212n2, 216n3
asymptomatic, 39, 99, 125, 152, 158. *See also* COVID infection
Aurelia, 79, 81, 206

Biden administration, 13, 166, 183, 184, 216n1, 216n2
Biden, Joe, 102, 213n8. *See also* Biden administration
binational families, 99. *See also* immigration status: mixed-status families
biomarkers, 5, 197
biosocial, 92–94
birth: companion, 91, 122, 145, 157; complications, 2, 41, 58, 69, 101, 135, 137, 147, 149, 214n11; negative experience, 7, 71–72, 81, 87, 127, 137, 144, 147, 154, 158–160; positive experience, 31, 133, 137–138, 140, 143, 147–149, 152, 158–160, 177, 188; premature, 67, 127; vacuum assisted, 41
birth center, 11, 139, 141, 163, 215n3. *See also* midwifery
birth certificate, 11–12, 46, 93, 163, 167. *See also* identity documents
birth control: access to, 57, 59–61, 65–66, 148–49; experimentation, 16, 30, 62; implant, 59; intrauterine device (IUD), 41, 51, 60–62, 161; long-acting reversible contraception (LARC), 61; pills, 161. *See also* obstetric experimentation

239

birth justice, 160. *See also* reproductive justice
birthright citizenship, 12, 17
blood pressure: emotional and social reference to, 28; high, 2, 41, 42, 51, 67–68, 73, 77, 79, 83, 89, 94, 105, 108, 110, 116, 136, 205; low, 104, 207. *See also* preeclampsia; *presión*
border crossing: card, 40, 73, 76, 122, 129, 144, 162–163; clandestine, 181, 183, 184; mobility in relation to, 15, 19; X-ray, 78
border health posts, disinfection stations, 14–15
border militarization, 12–14, 22, 69, 82, 86–88, 186, 190, 216n3
Border Patrol: agents, 1, 22, 74, 170, 181, 210n7, 212n2, 215n6; checkpoints, 25, 54, 64–65, 155, 170, 216n2; cross-border shootings involving, 22, helicopters and vehicles, 3, 74, 126, 170
border wait times, 78, 98, 212n2, 213n8
border wall, fence, 3, 28, 74, 126, 181
breastfeeding, 40–41, 50, 59, 66, 108, 110, 168–169, 176. *See also* lactation
breast pump, 108, 168, 176
Brisa, 1–6, 8–9, 19, 27–28, 31, 58, 110–112, 126–127, 134–137, 142–144, 159–160, 169–171, 178, 181, 192, 207, 215n1
bureaucratic disentitlement, 51
bureaucratic violence, 28–29, 47, 51, 114, 189

Camila, 146, 155–159
Castañeda, Heide, 15, 51
Celeste, 144, 215n6
Centers for Disease Control and Prevention (CDC), 13, 94, 191
Cerdeña, Jessica, 164
Chadwick, Rachelle, 28, 32. *See also* reproductive violence
Chavez, Leo, 12. *See also* anchor baby
childcare: pandemic closures affecting, 103, 114, 162, 164–66; reported challenges, 164, 168, 172, 176

child custody, 80, 115–16
Children's Health Insurance Program (CHIP) Perinatal, 8–10, 33, 39–40, 42–47, 51–54, 56–61, 65–66, 74, 92, 110–11, 113, 122, 131, 135–36, 142, 152, 160, 188, 191, 203, 204, 210n4, 211nn3, 4
child support, 115, 162, 167
Child Tax Credit, 149, 162, 179, 215n1
Cielo Vista Walmart, 21, 23, 124. *See also* mass shooting
community clinics, 33, 37, 52, 57, 142, 152, 192
conjugated harm, 118, 132–33, 164. *See also* conjugated oppression
conjugated oppression, 118, 214n1. *See also* conjugated harm
Coronavirus Aid, Relief, and Economic Security (CARES) Act, 25, 168, 210n8. *See also* COVID-19 pandemic: stimulus checks
cortisol: hair samples, 5, 33, 34, 99, 197, 198; in relation to preeclampsia, 199, 201, 213n9; metabolization, 200–201
COVID-19 infection: at time of birth, 39, 101, 103, 145, 155, 207; during pregnancy, 99, 101, 161. *See also* COVID-19 pandemic
COVID-19 pandemic: border closures, 24, 40, 68, 76–77, 119, 120–23, 130, 133, 162, 164–66, 179, 207; deaths, 23–24, 35, 41, 96, 100, 178, 184; Delta variant, 34, 173; fears, 35, 39, 41, 59, 101, 104, 118, 121–23, 125, 127, 173, 178, 206–7; hospital restrictions, 91, 108, 156; isolation, 39, 103, 121, 146, 161; Omicron variant, 34, 39, 150, 178; stay-at-home restrictions, 1, 58; stimulus checks, 102, 105, 168, 210n8; unemployment, 103, 105, 114, 116–17, 130, 161, 165, 171–72, 178, 210n8. *See also* Coronavirus Aid, Relief, and Economic Security (CARES) Act; COVID-19 infection

COVID-19 vaccine, hesitancy, 121, 173
cross-border relationship, 67. *See also* immigration: mixed-status families
C-section, 9, 35, 41, 61, 71, 91, 101, 108, 137, 138, 141, 144, 154, 157, 212n1, 214n11
Csordas, Thomas, 26. *See also* somatic modes of attention
cultural competency, 143, 215n5

Davis, Dána-Ain, 16, 30. *See also* obstetric racism
DDT, 14–15. *See also* Zyklon B
debt, 3, 6, 60, 169, 174, 178, 215n6
Deferred Action for Childhood Arrivals (DACA), 8, 56, 57, 102, 206
deportation: emotional toll from, 6, 12, 14, 26, 28, 55, 73, 77, 86, 87, 120, 170; physiological toll from, 28, 77, 79, 81, 87; racialized deportation projects, 20; under Trump administration, 12, 29, 86. *See also* Great Depression, deportation campaigns; somatic modes of attention
depression: antidepressants, 104; postpartum, 2, 7, 9, 40–41, 45, 49–50, 105, 135–36, 148–49, 152, 169, 206, 207
desesperación, symptoms, 1–4, 127. *See also* despair
despair, 1, 2, 4, 5, 6, 119, 127–28, 129, 153, 192. See also *desesperación*
detention: deaths in, 183; pregnant people in, 146
de Vos, Dieneke, 31. *See also* reproductive violence
diabetes: gestational diabetes, 2, 20, 27, 73, 83, 85, 101, 104, 109–10, 135, 204–7, 213n6; obesogens, 98, type 2, 41, 57, 84, 85, 101, 206
Diana, 114–120, 192
DiGeorge syndrome, 73
Dobbs v. Jackson, 185
doula: defined, 188; during COVID-19, 145; insurance coverage of, 189

eclampsia, 89–90, 112, 212n1, 213n3. *See also* preeclampsia
economic hardship, 1, 3, 14, 25, 41, 112, 115, 116, 121, 128, 167, 177, 179, 192
Eliana, 167–69, 178, 206
El Paso Convention Center, during COVID-19 pandemic, 24, 100
El Segundo Barrio, 126
embodiment, 26–27, 69–70, 86, 107
emergency room, 2, 8, 40, 55, 58, 90, 120, 134, 135, 152, 157, 160
empowerment, 190
endocrine disrupting chemicals, 98
endothelial dysfunction, 94, 213n9. *See also* preeclampsia
entrapment, 19, 54, 129
environmental contamination, 92, 98
environmental injustice, 92, 97, 112. *See also* American Smeltering and Refining Company (ASARCO); Smeltertown
epigenetics, 27, 102
eugenics, historical legacy, 16, 62, 139
explanatory models: Anahí, 72; Aurelia, 79; Brisa, 28; definition, 27, 70, 71, 85; Lina, 108; Marla, 79; Sofi, 76; Tamara, 81
extortion, 19, 183. *See also* narcoviolence

Fabiola, 121–24, 126
Families First Coronavirus Response Act, 41
Family and Medical Leave Act (FMLA), 109, 161, 178
family separation: due to extended border closure, 179, 207; due to immigration policies, 13, 78, 123, 192
Farfán-Santos, Elizabeth, 43. *See also* womb-body divide
Farmer, Paul, 187. *See also* pragmatic solidarity
Federally Qualified Health Centers (FQHCs), 142, 215n4

federal poverty level (FPL), 43, 44, 165, 210n2, 211n2, 211n6
fertility, hyperfertility, 15
fetal breathing movements, 150
fetal personhood, 43
Flor, 58
food insecurity, 102, 117–18, 130, 132, 205–7. See also food pantry
food pantry, 33, 115, 117. See also food insecurity
food stamps, 55, 73, 115, 117, 148, 162. See also Supplemental Nutrition Assistance Program (SNAP)
formula feeding: hesitancy, 108, 168, 169, 176; shortage, 166–67, 176
Fort Bliss, 132
Frederick, Angela, 153

George W. Bush administration, 11, 43
Geronimus, Arline, 85. See also weathering
gestational diabetes, 2, 20, 27, 73, 83, 85, 101, 104, 109–10, 135, 204–7, 213n6
Great Depression, deportation campaigns, 11, 140. See also deportation
green card, 10, 40
gun control, 4, 6

harassment, 71, 170
Harthorn, Barbara Herr, 111
headache, 2, 51, 89. See also hypertensive crisis
Healthy Texas Women (HTW), 45, 59, 60
Helena, 128–129
HELLP syndrome, 90. See also preeclampsia
hemorrhage, postpartum, 2, 135, 147, 206, 207, 213n2
high-risk: pregnancy, 83; provider, 153, 154, 155
Hispanic invasion, 12, 21. See also birthright citizenship; mass shooting
Horton, Sarah, 24

Houchen Settlement House, 140. See also midwifery
humanitarian parole, 183
hydrocephaly, 63–64, 207
hypertension, 9, 91, 96, 99, 110, 112, 205, 213n2, 214n15
hypertensive crisis, 51, 89. See also headache

iatrogenic harm, 30, 137
identity documents, 3, 12, 163, 170. See also birth certificate
Immigration and Customs Enforcement (ICE), 115, 146
immigration: concerns, 4–5, 25, 32, 36–37, 68–70, 72, 77, 82, 87, 112, 117, 120, 133, 179, 186, 205–7; first-generation, 33; raids, 12, 87; reform, 10–11, 102, 190; second-generation, 4, 5, 33, 70, 79, 81; targeted enforcement, 87; trends, 19. See also cross-border relationship; Zero Tolerance
immigration status: adjustment of, 10, 53, 54, 75, 83, 175; children of immigrants, 12; mixed-status families, 8, 29, 78, 81, 117; naturalization, 10, 24, 52; permanent residency, 8, 19, 43, 53–54, 57, 59, 67, 70, 73, 75–76, 81–82, 119, 122–24, 129, 166, 170–71, 203–5, 207, 210n7; precarious, 3, 5, 8, 23, 29, 72–73, 92, 171, 177; undocumented, 1, 3, 8–9, 12, 22, 25–26, 45, 56, 60–61, 67, 70, 73–75, 78–82, 86, 99, 102, 112, 115, 120, 127–28, 144, 149, 203–7, 210n8, 216n2. See also binational families
impotencia. See *impotente*
impotente, 2, 37, 82, 161, 164, 177. See also powerlessness
induction, labor, 71, 90, 101, 106, 135, 138, 154, 157, 158, 214n13
infant death, 7, 17, 19, 140, 166, 176, 191, 205, 211n4

infant mortality. *See* infant death
inflation, 176, 178, 183, 185
interdisciplinary research, 5, 34, 198
intimate partner violence, 53, 74, 207
Iris, 176, 178
Isabela, 21, 23, 124–26, 192, 207
Itzel, 11–12, 161–65, 168, 172, 177, 179, 192, 207

Janeth, 100, 104–5, 110, 112–13, 206
Jazmine, 47–51, 146–49, 159–60, 175
Jim Crow laws, 139
Julia, 82–83, 85, 206

kinship, 70, 79, 81, 84, 181
Kleinman, Arthur, 71. *See also* explanatory models
Krieger, Nancy, 20

labor augmentation, 137, 138, 150, 151, 157, 158
lactation, 39, 210n1. *See also* breastfeeding
language barriers, 151
Latina Health Paradox, 19, 46, 77
Laverty, Ciara, 31. *See also* reproductive violence
lead, contamination, 97
legal violence, 28–32, 51, 189
likely public charge, 9–10, 52–54, 144, 210n4
Liliana, 57–60, 174–75, 178, 207
Lina, 17–19, 63–64, 100, 105–8, 146, 153–55, 158–59, 175, 207
local biologies, 26–27, 69–70, 85–86, 88, 95, 120, 186
López, Iris, 61
Lorena, 56
low birthweight, 7, 20, 23. *See also* birth: premature
Lupe, 89–91, 100, 108–10, 113, 176–77, 206
Lydia, 73, 76–77

MacDorman, Marian, 7. *See also* maternal mortality
Magdalena, 61
magnesium sulfate, 91, 213n2
maquiladoras, 98, 108, 213n7
Margot, 61, 73–74, 76–77, 87, 205
Marla, 67–68, 70, 77–79, 81, 86–87, 205
mass shooting: anxiety after, 23, 35, 124, 192, 207; El Paso, 21, 23; racially motivated, 4, 22, 124, 184. *See also* Cielo Vista Walmart; Hispanic invasion
mastitis, 39, 40, 66, 152, 160, 207
maternal health outcomes, adverse, 4, 19, 21, 23, 27, 28, 30, 32, 56, 66, 71, 72, 79, 87, 88, 90, 188
maternal morbidity, 2, 20, 45, 46, 66, 90, 112, 191
maternal mortality, 7, 45, 83, 90
maternity ward, 16, 139, 140, 141, 215n7
Mavuso, Mary-Jane Jace, 28, 32. *See also* reproductive violence
Medicaid: Emergency, 45, 110, 136, 191, 211n2, 211n4; expiration, 41–42, 48–51, 55, 60–61, 126, 142, 148–49; extension, 44–46, 49–50, 66, 187, 209n3, 211n2; for pregnant women, 8, 33, 42–48, 55, 90, 104, 110, 125, 154, 187–88, 191, 203–4, 209n2, 211n2; public health emergency, 41–42, 46, 48–49, 66, 105, 114, 185; renewal, 48–50, 55
medical experimentation. *See* birth control: experimentation
medical negligence, 65, 136
medical racism: Chinese immigrants, 10; Mexican laborers, 10
medical records, 20, 33, 46, 77, 110, 111, 116, 197, 213n4, 214n12
Medically Underserved Area (MUA), 120
medicalization, overmedicalization, 137
Menjívar, Cecilia, 72. *See also* immigration status: precarious

midwifery: birth registrations with midwives, 11; Black midwives, 138; Certified Nurse Midwife (CNM), 31, 44, 139, 188; Certified Professional Midwife (CPM), 139; credentialing, 138, 140; professionalization, 138–39, 141; shortage, 149, 152, 159, 188; smear campaigns, 138; training, 137–38, 140–42, 159, 188. *See also* birth center; Houchen Settlement House
mifepristone, 64, 185
Migrant Protection Protocols, 13
misoprostol, 64
Morales, Cristina, 21. *See also* state-sponsored violence
Murillo, Lina-Maria, 62

narcoviolence, 19, 80, 212n3. *See also* extortion; War on Drugs
National Guard, 14, 100, 126, 182, 184
neonatal intensive care unit (NICU), 145, 152, 155
nervios, 73, 74, 124. *See also* anxiety; panic
neural tube defect, 106–8. *See also* spina bifida; Texas Neural Tube Defect Project
Ngai, Mae, 12. *See also* alien citizens
North American Free Trade Agreement (NAFTA), 98
Novak, Nicole, 20

Oaks, Laury, 111
obesity, 91, 96, 98, 102, 110–11
OB-GYN (doctor of obstetrics and gynecology), model of birth, 137, 151, 159
obstetric experimentation, 16, 30. *See also* birth control: experimentation
obstetric racism, 16, 30. *See also* obstetric violence
obstetric violence, 29–31, 58, 136, 143, 144, 160. *See also* obstetric racism
oil fields, 59, 174, 175

Operation Border Health Preparedness, 14. *See also* Operation Lone Star
Operation Lone Star, 14. *See also* Operation Border Health Preparedness
Organista, Kurt, 3. See also *desesperación*
Ortega, Lina, 49
oxidative stress, 94, 213n9

Page Act of 1875, 10
Pandemic Unemployment Assistance (PUA), 114, 161
panic, 2, 116, 119, 121, 122, 124, 157, 158, 177. See also *nervios*
parental leave, 35, 36, 168, 172, 178, 189
passport: denial, 11, 163; phenotypic, 15
perpetual foreignness, 11, 14, 19
Piñeda, Richard, 22
Pitocin, 151, 157, 158
placenta: accreta, 206, 214n11; implantation, 90, 93; manual removal of, 2, 135, 147, 207; retained, 2, 135, 147
ports of entry, 14, 119, 124, 212n2
Porvenir Massacre (1918), 22
powerlessness, 1, 3, 164. See also *impotencia*; *impotente*
prenatal care: delayed initiation of, 50, 126; underutilization of, 10
pragmatic solidarity, 187
Pregnancy Risk Assessment Monitoring System (PRAMS), 47, 94, 191
preeclampsia: and COVID-19, 92, 95–96, 99–105, 213n10, 214n12; mortality, 90, 109, 213n6; nitrogen dioxide, 98; postpartum, 2, 8, 100, 108–10, 113, 136, 169, 206, 214n14; prevalence, 37, 110. *See also* blood pressure: high; eclampsia; endocrine disrupting chemicals; endothelial dysfunction; HELLP syndrome
presión, 27–28. *See also* blood pressure: high; hypertension
private health insurance, 8, 56–57, 142, 154
promatoras, 192

public health emergency, 13, 41–42, 46, 48–49, 66, 105, 114, 148, 181, 183–85, 216n3

racialization, 14
racism: medical, 10, 30; racist imagery, 12; systemic, 92
Rebecca, 60
Remain in Mexico, 13, 181. *See* Title 42
reproductive habitus, 74
reproductive injustice, 32
reproductive justice, 31–32, 37, 43, 47, 160, 172, 179, 185–90. *See also* birth justice
reproductive violence, 4, 28–32, 65, 87, 133, 160, 179, 186–87
resiliency, 119, 177
respiratory distress, 68, 205
risk: discourse, 16, 83, 96, 111; individualized, 91–92, 111; maternal, 69, 109, 118
Rita, 9, 205
Roberts, James, 93. *See also* preeclampsia
Rodriguez, Maria, 211n4
Roe v. Wade, 25, 62–63. *See also* abortion
Romo, David, 14. *See also* Zyklon B
Rosas, Gilberto, 22

Saldaña-Tejeda, Abril, 96, 111
Salma, 41–42, 47–48, 54–56, 84–85, 206
Sandra, 57, 100–104, 110, 112, 171–72, 177–79, 206
Sara, 53–54
Sinclair, Heather, 139
Singer, Merrill, 96. *See also* syndemic interactions
Smeltertown, 97. *See also* environmental injustice
social epidemiology, 26
social support, 3, 120, 130–31, 178
Sofi, 74–76, 205
somatic modes of attention, 26. *See also* deportation
sonogram, 53, 63, 155, 156

spina bifida: maternal folic acid, 107; meningocele, 106. *See also* neural tube defect
substance abuse, 45
suicidal thoughts, 60, 104–5, 113, 157, 206
Supplemental Nutrition Assistance Program (SNAP), 117, 185. *See also* food stamps
surveillance, reproductive control, 16
Susana, 60
state-sponsored violence, 21–22
sterilization, forced, 28, 30, 61, 190
stratified access, 42, 46–47, 57–58
stratified livability, 25
stress: acute, 86–87, 92, 212n4; chronic, 69, 85–87, 92, 94, 99, 102, 212n4; cumulative, 85, 95, 110; physiology, 26–28; response, 26–28, 69, 86, 94, 102; stress-sensitive health outcomes, 5, 72, 85
structural competency, 143, 159–60, 188, 215n5
structural racism, 16, 17, 30
structural vulnerability, 118, 119, 190
syndemic interactions, 96, 105, 110
systemic inflammation, 94

tachycardia, 156
Talia, 131–32, 207
Tamara, 80–81, 87, 205
temporary zone of inclusion, 8
Texas Health and Human Services (HHS), 42, 48–50, 115
Texas House Bill-133 (HB-133), 45–46
Texas Maternal Mortality and Morbidity Taskforce, 7, 45
Texas Neural Tube Defect Project, 107. *See also* neural tube defect
Texas Rangers, 22
Texas Workforce Commission, 114
Title 42, 13, 24, 181–84, 216nn1–2, 216n3. *See also* Remain in Mexico
Title X clinics, 45, 211n5
toxicology paradigm, 96
transborder. *See* transfronterizo
transfronterizo, 17

Treaty of Hidalgo (1848), 14
Tricare, 56
Trump administration, 9–13, 24, 33, 52–53, 86, 126, 163, 186, 212n2, 216n1
Trump, Donald. *See* Trump administration

unemployment benefits, 102, 105, 114, 116–17, 161, 165, 171–72, 178–79, 210n8
uninsured, 7–8, 51, 55–56, 125, 136, 203–4
United States Citizenship and Immigration Services (USCIS), 9, 40
University Medical Center (UMC), 116, 135–36, 141–45, 159
urinary tract infection (UTI), 9
US-born citizens, 1, 5, 11–12, 33, 41, 53, 64, 67, 72, 106, 155, 163, 203–7
US State Department, 11, 163

Veronica, 53
Violence Against Women Act (VAWA), 53, 75, 205, 207

Wahlberg, Ayo, 25. *See also* stratified livability
War on Drugs, 80, 212n3. *See also* narcoviolence
weathering, 85
welfare reform, 10–11
Willen, Sarah, 26
William Beaumont Army Medical Center, 141
womb-body divide, 43–44
Women, Infants, and Children (WIC), 9–10, 40, 52, 162, 166–67, 210n1
World Health Organization (WHO), 149

Yolanda, 130–32

Zahra, 73, 205
Zavella, Patricia, 186
Zero Tolerance, 13, 186. *See also* immigration
Zyklon B, 14. *See also* DDT

ABOUT THE AUTHOR

CARINA HECKERT is Associate Professor of Anthropology in the Department of Sociology and Anthropology at the University of Texas at El Paso.

www.ingramcontent.com/pod-product-compliance
Lightning Source LLC
Chambersburg PA
CBHW031146020426
42333CB00013B/527